Adrenal Insufficiency Workbook

A daily diary for you, your doctor, and your family

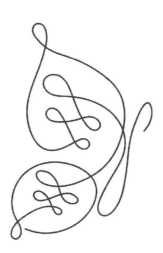

By
Lisa C. Baker, RNHP, CNC

© 2019 Lisa C. Baker

10 9 8 7 6 5 4 3 2 1

ISBN 9781794402225

Disclaimer
This book is not intended as a substitute for the medical advice of physicians. The reader should regularly consult a physician in matters relating to his/her health and particularly with respect to any symptoms that may require diagnosis or medical attention.

Published by
Third Childhood Publishing
PO Box 750471
Topeka, KS 750471

Purpose of This Book

As an Adrenal Insufficiency patient, I have found myself trying to put together stacks of notes, snippets of paper, and remembering things to tell my endocrinologist when I 'finally' get in. I never have it all together. When visiting other, or new, doctors, I always have to explain my situation over and over and recite symptoms and answer questions even though I've been diagnosed for almost forever!, then put together a format in a notebook so I could just keep everything on place where I could just grab it and go whenever I had an appointment.

As I began working on my Naturopathic internship, I started using my own case for study. I started adding fields for additional information that I knew would help my studies. Gradually, I started noticing trends in things that may lead up to crisis or pre-crisis, and symptoms I didn't even realize I was having because I could now see the trends in black and white. This also helped my doctor help me – I could call or visit when certain problems were creeping up, and we could attack them early on and hopefully avoid crisis and extra stress on my body.

If you keep this book up to date, it will be useful for you in the above ways, but also for your family, paramedics or other emergency personnel. Just grab the book every time you have an appointment and you have all of you notes to discuss. Just grab this book everytime you have a new doctor – they may even want to photocopy it! And if you need emergency intervention, your family can give the personnel this book so they can see not only your history, but events leading right up to the incident.

If you miss a day, it's ok. But don't do it too often!

I hope you find this helpful in determining ways to avoid emergency situations, and ways to help yourself. I also hope that this helps you in communicating with doctors and emergency personnel.

Be happy and enjoy life, one day at a time!

My History and Facts

YOU IDENTIFY WITH *yourself.there are* THINGS YOU WANT TO *experience and other* THINGS THAT YOU WANT *To avoid.*

- Frederick Lenz

Make this as complete as possible, so that in the event you are unable to communicate with emergency personnel, their questions can be answered. It also makes finding triggers, trends, and helpful tips more obvious and make sense! Use pencil for items that may change frequently. If you can't fit all of the information in, there is a space at the end of the questionnaire for Additional Information. Just put an asterisk (*) in the space to indicate looking in the Additional Comments section.

Full Legal Name_____

Physical Address_____

_____

Mailing address_____

_____

My phone #_____ **My e-mail**_____

Emergency Contacts

Name_____ Ph. #_____

Name_____ Ph. #_____

Name_____ Ph. #_____

My primary physician name _____

Primary physician phone _____ **PP e-mail**_____

My insurance company _____

    Policy Holder Name_____

    Policy Number_____

    Phone Number_____

Do I work? Yes_____ Hahaha_____

Where?_____

Occupation _____

My occupations throughout life _____

_____

My diagnoses
    Diagnosis_____

    _____

    Date diagnosed_____

    Symptoms that led to diagnosis_____

    _____

    _____

    _____

    Triggers_____

    _____

    _____

    _____

Current treatment_____

_____

_____

_____

_____

Drug allergies

    Drug_____**Symptoms/Warnings**_____

    Drug_____**Symptoms/Warnings**_____

    Drug_____**Symptoms/Warnings**_____

    Drug_____**Symptoms/Warnings**_____

    Drug_____**Symptoms/Warnings**_____

Food allergies

    Food_____**Symptoms/Warnings**_____

    Food_____**Symptoms/Warnings**_____

    Food_____**Symptoms/Warnings**_____

    Food_____**Symptoms/Warnings**_____

    Food_____**Symptoms/Warnings**_____

Physical limitations_____

_____

_____

Past surgeries

    Procedure_____**Date**_____**Where**_____

    Procedure_____**Date**_____**Where**_____

    Procedure_____**Date**_____**Where**_____

    Procedure_____**Date**_____**Where**_____

    Procedure_____**Date**_____**Where**_____

Current List of Medications

      (See the beginning of each month in the diary. Meds and supplements are updated each month for the purposes of this workbook.)

*Additional Comments:

_____

_____

_____

_____

_____

_____

_____

_____

_____

_____

_____

_____

_____

_____

Information for Friends and Family

So someone you care about has Adrenal Insufficiency. What does that mean to you??

It means you need to be there for not only support, but in a medical emergency. It means you need to check on them, as well as be ready to provide any respite care for their caregivers. Check on the caregivers, too! And it also means you need to have important information at the ready, should medical personnel be in need of this information. Particularly if you are a family member, coworker, or anyone else who cares about an AI patient, or has the opportunity to spend time around them.

Even if you are not in the same home, or even the same town, the information you have allows you to not only check on the patient and the caregiver, but to provide the same information to emergency personnel should that be necessary.

This booklet provides an easy to understand look at why this is important, what things are important to understand and know, and emergency procedures. It does not give you deep medical information, but does provide references and resources should you be so inclined to learn more about the physiology of AI.

The most important thing to remember is this:
Cortisol and Aldosterone are NECESSARY FOR HUMAN LIFE. With inadequate quantities, or little of one or both, the patient's body will NOT be able to function and shock, coma and death will occur.

Why is this such a big deal?

So, let's say you know somebody with Diabetes. You know a few things about that, such as you don't ever offer them things with sugar in it (and hopefully no starches and carbs!), and if they say they need their insulin shot, you jump and do whatever is needed to make sure they get their shot. Even though you don't know why, you know they could go into a coma, and could die. If they start shaking, or begin acting confused or angry, you ask them if they need to eat something. You care, and don't want them to die.

Or, let's say you know somebody with a heart condition. They grab their heart, yours jumps, too. You ask them if they need a pill under their tongue. You try and keep bad news from them, try not to upset them, and ask others to do the same thing. You don't know the 'whys,' but you know they could die.

How do you react to your relative or co-worker with Adrenal Insufficiency? Please do not get angry when they are confused or irrational.... Know that it is a medical symptom and a sign they need help. Please do not ignore them when they say they are tired or feel sick or faint, these are signs they could be going into an Adrenal Crisis.

It is important to know that they could die, too, and very quickly.

Let's break down Adrenal Insufficiency in a laymen's format, so you can understand what is happening to your family member or friend, and so you know how important it is to respond.

Adrenal Hormone Roles

The Adrenal glands are part of the body's Endocrine System. You've heard of some of the other glands – the pituitary, the thyroid, even the ovaries and testicles. The Endocrine System is a tricky mechanism, and is a bit like playing dominoes. Something goes wrong with one of them, and it affects all of the ones after it. So, since the Adrenal glands come pretty far down in the chain, the reason they go awry can lie in several other glands or problems.

Although Addison's Disease usually occurs later in life as a result of injury to the adrenal glands (for various reasons), or overuse of steroids for other medical reasons, it is non-curable and requires lifelong steroid (and possibly mineralocorticoid) replacement to sustain life. The other cause of Adrenal Insufficiency is Congenital Adrenal Hyperplasia. This is something the person is born with, and there is no cure for. There are varying enzyme deficiencies which cause it, and some forms of it can cause death shortly after birth if not diagnosed, while other forms do not 'onset' until late puberty. The illness requires lifelong steroid (and sometimes mineralocorticoid) replacement to sustain life.

There are also patients who have had adrenal or pituitary gland removed, so therefore, they make NO steroids or mineralocorticoids at all and MUST have lifelong replacement, or die.

Sometimes, patients can be overmedicated with steroids and develop Cushing's Syndrome (not to be confused by Cushing's Disease which is usually caused by a tumor). Cushing's Syndrome is developed from having too much steroid in the body for too long. and is the complete opposite of Adrenal Insufficiency.

So what are these steroid and mineralocorticoid hormones??

Some people think when you speak of a disease with the Adrenal Glands, the only hormone involved is Adrenaline. In fact, Adrenaline is not an issue with Adrenal Insufficiency.

The steroid (glucocorticoid) is "Cortisol." What does cortisol do?
Cortisol is a life-sustaining hormone. Cortisol helps regulate blood sugar, metabolism, the immune system, heart and blood vessels, and central nervous system activation, to name a few. When a person's body is stressed either physically or emotionally, cortisol is extremely important and is what keeps us alive during these times.

STRESS. That needs more explanation.

Stress is such a buzz word lately. We are not talking about mortgage due-car payment late-kids are sick kind of stress; although that WILL affect your cortisol levels, and greatly. But stress includes physiological stress. Stress on the body from illness, such as a cold, fever, injury, headache, physical labor, running, etc. During a stressful event, your cortisol levels multiply up to 10x. If your body does not make enough cortisol for normal function of your body, you have to replace it. Then, if you face a stressful situation – whether it is something listed above, or even an argument with a loved one, you need to take way more medication than you normally would take to make up for the 10x increase your body cannot make. If you cannot do this, you will collapse and could possibly die. You just don't have enough cortisol, and the circulatory system starts shutting down. It is similar to a gas tank running on fumes. You may have enough gas to get to the corner station, but if a dog runs out in front of you and you have to step on it and swerve, you may use all of what you have left up in an instant. And then the car dies.

The mineralocorticoid mentioned is called "Aldosterone." If you have high blood pressure, you may have heard of Aldosterone, as it is oftentimes the cause if you have too much. But with Adrenal Insufficiency, you have hardly any, or none at all. Patients with Primary Addison's normally suffer from what is know as "Salt Wasting" and do not have enough Aldosterone. The most common form of Congenital Adrenal Hyperplasia is due to an enzyme deficiency called 21-Hydroxylase, and is nicknamed "Salt Wasting CAH." These patients have hardly enough, if any, Aldosterone. What does Aldosterone do??

Aldosterone regulates blood pressure, salt and water balance in the body, and potassium. Without enough Aldosterone, a patient's blood pressure can drop very quickly to shock state. Without having enough salt, the patient can become seriously dehydrated. Along with dehydration, the body starts shutting down. All systems start shutting down until the patient reaches circulatory collapse (SHOCK), when the only thing left is the heart circulating blood and the kidneys barely assisting in the blood circulation. Once the patient reaches this state, it is a life threatening event. Only emergency intervention can save the patient's life.

It must be stressed that these are just short, cursory, laymen explanations and there is much, much more involved in these processes, and the symptoms and consequences are many times more.

Medication

To replace cortisol, patients are placed on Hydrocortisone, Prednisone, or Dexamethasone. Hydrocortisone (or HC) is the medication of choice for Primary and Secondary Addison's Disease, and Dexamethasone is the medication of choice for Congenital Adrenal Hyperplasia, although there are variations due to severity and tolerance. The dosage is usually several times a day, oftentimes mimicking the body's own rhythm of how it makes cortisol naturally, with additional doses needed in times of physiological and emotional stress. In the event of an Adrenal Crisis, an emergency injection of Solu-Cortef or Dexamethasone is needed immediately, even if the patient is being transported to the ER. Do not wait for the Emergency Room, this could cost a person their life.

Some patients also take herbal adaptogens to help regulate cortisol – IF they produce any amount of cortisol on their own. If there is none produced, of course, it can't be leveled. Some patients also take homeopathic cortisol instead of the above referenced pharmaceuticals, should they happen to be a patient of a naturopath or integrative medicine physician. An emergency injection is still prescribed and recommended.

To replace Aldosterone, patients are prescribed Fludrocortisone (brand name Florinef). There is no other medication, nor is there any herbal or homeopathic medication to assist with increasing Aldosterone production and levels. However, some patients are able to keep their sodium and electrolyte levels normal by taking salt tablets, using extra salt (sea salt and pink Himalayan salt are most recommended), electrolyte replacements, etc. In the event of an impending Adrenal Crisis, or if the patient feels dehydrated or faint, immediate salt ingestion is usually called for.

Things to be careful about

Adrenal Insufficiency patients need to be very careful about many things, including:

•Being around sick people. Most AI patients have very low immune systems, and can get ill very, very quickly and easily. Any illness requires more cortisol in the body (up to 10x as much as normal), and if the patient doesn't 'dose up' in time, can find themselves nearing an Adrenal Crisis. In addition, vomiting and diarrhea can cause quick dehydration, and an almost guaranteed Adrenal Crisis. Extra cortisol is needed for the physiological stress of any illness.

•Injuries also require extra cortisol, fast.

•Emotional stress causes just as much usage of available cortisol and the need for extra cortisol as physiological stress.

•Heat and Humidity. Both contribute to dehydration and impending Adrenal Crisis in patients that are salt wasting.

•Over exertion. For the same reasons as above.

•Fever.

Adrenal Insufficiency patients should always wear a medical alert bracelet stating "Steroid Dependent," "Adrenal Insufficiency" or other identifiers. They should also carry wallet cards with not only their dosage instructions, but their doctor's contact information. If your loved one does not have either, encourage them to obtain them.

Signs to watch for

When the Adrenal Insufficiency patient starts feeing confused, emotional, fatigued, tired, ill, etc., these are signs that cortisol and/or aldosterone is out of balance and the patient requires medication. Actual staggering, vomiting, diarrhea and fainting require emergency injections. By the time a person faints, their body has shut down almost to the coma stage.

Low Blood Pressure. If the patient has LOW blood pressure, immediate medical assistance is needed.

Fever. Fever requires 'stress dosing' levels (extra doses to cover what the body would normally make in response to physiological stress of fever).

When to offer assistance

If you see any of the signs shown above, intervene and make sure the patient has taken extra medication to cover the needs of the body. If the patient is vomiting, has diarrhea or is staggering and confused, get them to sit down or stabilize in one place, and help them receive their emergency injection. Know where it is!! Sometimes the patient cannot remember what is is, or even where it is, when confused and the body is shutting down. Failure to emergency inject and follow up is a life threatening situation.

If you offer a salt wasting patient water, be sure you also include electrolytes and/or salt. Electrolytes are available as drops and even tablets to add to water. Not all commercially bottled waters which are labeled as 'electrolyte enhanced' contain sodium (salt), the ONE electrolyte salt wasters need!! Make sure you know which ones are appropriate, or read the labels.

Adrenal Crisis

When a patient exhibits signs of an Adrenal Crisis, immediate medical assistance is needed, or coma and subsequent death can quickly occur. In addition, irreversible damage can occur leaving handicaps and life altering affects without timely intervention.

Adrenal crisis signs are vomiting, diarrhea, confusion, lethargy, muscle twitching, irritability, dehydration and fainting. Not all patients have all symptoms, and some patients have other symptoms. Get to know your loved one's normal symptoms for Adrenal Crisis so you can help save their life. Emergency injection administration is needed immediately, along with an ambulance or being taken to the Emergency Room if it is close enough

Studies show that even with proper medication and management, Adrenal Insufficiency patients can expect Adrenal Crises. Not all patients experience them often, and some more frequently than others. But the patient is always a few steps away from one at any given time, and as a caregiver or someone who is around an AI patient, you must be alert to the signs and know where their medication is.

If you are not knowledgeable about the ins and outs of Adrenal Insufficiency – and nobody expects you to be! – PLEASE make sure you at least tell ANY person in authority wherever you are, that the person is STEROID DEPENDENT. They may not know what that means, either, but they are the people able to communicate to medical personnel the immediate and life sustaining information needed to save the patient's life. If your diabetic friend went into a coma, you would certainly tcll thosc in authority they were insulin dependent, or you'd tell a possible heart attack victim that they have a heart condition. Please do the same for your AI loved one.

After the Crisis
Just as it sometimes takes weeks or days to decline into an Adrenal Crisis, it often takes days and weeks to recover from one; time for the body to gather enough cortisol and aldosterone to function normally, with the aid of constant medication, electrolytes, rest, etc. If hospitalization is needed, the doctor will keep the patient until they are stabilized. If an emergency room visit is all that is necessary and the patient is released, immediate care will be more intense. Although the patient will seem exceptionally well if they have had emergency cortisol injections or placed in their IV, this is a reaction to the medication. Do not expect them to be able to walk, think, or perform any functions in a normal manner for quite some time (10 to 14 days is not abnormal). In fact, encouraging them to do so could put them in another life threatening situation very quickly. Remember the analogy of the Diabetic or Heart patient. You would not expect someone recovering from a diabetic seizure or coma, or a heart attack, to be able to be 'up to par' for quite sometime. Respect their cane, walker, or handicap permit if they have one – this is the time they really need it!

Make sure you check on them, and let them know you care about them. This cannot be stressed enough! A person who has had an Adrenal Crisis was minutes, maybe an hour, from dying. Let them know you care. Find out if you can run errands for them, handle any situations or business matters, go to the store, prepare food, and make sure they have their medication. If they are sleeping a lot, check on them often to ensure they are not in crisis while sleeping. And if they have a caregiver, PLEASE check on that person often, too. They need respite services, and for people to be concerned about them, too. It is quite stressful to care for a loved one who may go into an Adrenal Crisis at any time.

Things NOT to do
•Do NOT get the patient angry, upset, or intentionally put them into situations that are stressful. That is like giving a diabetic sugar.

•Do NOT expose them to sick people. With little or no immune system, the consequences could be devastating.

•Do NOT call them lazy. It is not that they are lazy, but are physically INCAPABLE of doing many things if the cortisol and aldosterone levels are not adequate. You would not get mad at an amputee for not running, right?

•Do NOT say things such as:

"You don't LOOK sick?!"
Usually they don't, unless their medication is off. Diabetics and heart patients don't look sick, either. For some reason, people tend to think that in order to be sick, one must be in the hospital, wearing a gown, be in a wheelchair, or crippled. Fact is, a person with AI could have an Adrenal Crisis at any time, and every single day has to watch their medication, their activities, food, climate, etc., in order to prevent one.

"You're too young to be sick."
Huh? There are AI patients who were BORN with Congenital Adrenal Hyperplasia – that's what Congenital means. There are children out there with cancer, in wheelchairs, and other illnesses. NOBODY is too young to be sick.

"Everyone gets tired."
'Tired' is just a SYMPTOM of AI. It is something that must be heeded, and means they need to slow down, or need to stress dose with their medication, or they could be heading for an Adrenal Crisis. Being tired is just a symptom, and just one of MANY. Being tired is not the worst part of AI, but the fact that your body cannot handle illness, stress, exertion, heat, and can't control blood pressure, etc. are way more serious than being tired. If you think an AI patient only has issues with being tired, PLEASE re-read this booklet, and further educate yourself about AI.

"You're Just Having a Bad Day."
This might be true. And all the more reason to be concerned. Make sure that they are upping, or stress dosing with their medication, and you check on them. A bad day, which everyone has, can turn into their 'last day' very quickly.

"Everybody has stress."
Of course they do. And most everybody (those without AI) have enough cortisol and aldosterone for their body to deal with it without shutting down.

You get the picture.

Instead, tell them you care about them, you love them, they can count on you, etc. That's what any person deserves and wants.

Lastly
Remember that you don't need to know all of the physiological ins and outs of Adrenal Insufficiency, unless you want to. What you DO need to know is:
•This is a life threatening illness.
•Where the patient's emergency medication is (even if you are not there, but are able to tell somebody).
•What to tell persons in authority – that the patient is STEROID DEPENDENT. This is not only important because it will save their life, but STOPPING steroids without proper 'weaning' can cause a life or death situation, as well.
•That the person does not need to be around sick people, or stressful situations, or put into exerting situations.
•That they need support, as do their caregivers.

Stress-Relieving Doodle Page

Data Entry

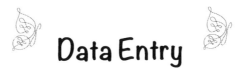

The following pages are for you to keep your Diary – these entries will
- be useful in determining trends
- be helpful during your doctor's appointments
- an extremely useful 'take-along' should you need emergency assistance
- helpful to any caretaker or family member when attempting to get help or just to understand

You may label each month so you can start at any time during the calendar year. If you miss a day here and there, that's ok – just don't make a regular habit of it! Use a dark pencil or a black pen in case your doctor or the hospital wishes to make photocopies.

On a daily basis, you will be tracking:

- *Blood Pressure*
    This can be helpful in knowing early when you may need salt, are becoming dehydrated, and assist in preventing a crisis by reversing the situation. It is also helpful to your doctor to assess fludrocortisone or steroid dosage, as well as becoming aware of how certain events, activities, new medication, and certain foods can affect you.

- *Pulse*
    This is helpful when evaluating along with Blood Pressure and is very important!

- *Blood Sugar/Glucose*
    This is important to some people who may be diabetic or hypoglycemic, but it is also helpful in evaluating cortisol levels or dosage of steroids. Often, cortisol is known to coincide with glucose numbers. Too low of glucose can mean low cortisol. Too much steroid replacement can lead to high blood sugar. This is also helpful information to a physician who is evaluating you for possible pre- or diabetes. Often used by AI patients to confirm if they feel a crisis is coming, or they feel their steroid dosage is too high. NEVER CHANGE MEDICATION DOSAGE WITHOUT CONSULTING YOUR ENDOCRINOLOGIST. Take this record to her for proper advice!

- *Menstrual Cycle status*

- *Daily activities and stressors*

- *How do you 'feel'?*

- *Food and hydration*

- *Medicine and supplement changes, lab reports, etc*

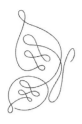

Month & Year

As of the first of the month, I am currently taking the following medications:

Name   Dosage   Frequency

_____   _____   _____

_____   _____   _____

_____   _____   _____

_____   _____   _____

_____   _____   _____

_____   _____   _____

_____   _____   _____

I have the following Dr. appointments and procedures scheduled:

_____

_____

_____

I have the following non-standard activities planned:

_____

_____

_____

DATE_____

Blood Pressure   sitting ____/____   standing ____/____   Pulse _____BPM

Blood Sugar _____   **Menstrual cycle phase**   __pre   __pms   __have period

Today I physically feel:

_____

_____

*Today I mentally feel:*_____

_____

Any unusual activity or events: _____

_____

Food & Hydration:_____

_____

_____

_____

Medical appointments, procedures or notes: _____

_____

DATE_____

Blood Pressure   sitting ____/____   standing ____/____   Pulse _____BPM

Blood Sugar _____   **Menstrual cycle phase**   __pre   __pms   __have period

Today I physically feel:

_____

_____

*Today I mentally feel:*_____

_____

Any unusual activity or events: _____

_____

Food & Hydration:_____

_____

_____

_____

Medical appointments, procedures or notes: _____

_____

DATE_____

Blood Pressure sitting ____/____ standing ____/____ Pulse _____BPM

Blood Sugar _____   **Menstrual cycle phase** __pre __pms __have period

Today I physically feel:

_____

_____

*Today I mentally feel:*_____

_____

Any unusual activity or events: _____

_____

Food & Hydration:_____

_____

_____

_____

Medical appointments, procedures or notes: _____

_____

DATE_____

Blood Pressure   sitting ____/____   standing ____/____   Pulse _____BPM

Blood Sugar _____   **Menstrual cycle phase** __pre __pms __have period

Today I physically feel:

_____

_____

*Today I mentally feel:*_____

_____

Any unusual activity or events: _____

_____

Food & Hydration:_____

_____

_____

_____

Medical appointments, procedures or notes: _____

_____

DATE_____

Blood Pressure sitting ____/____ standing ____/____ Pulse _____BPM

Blood Sugar _____ **Menstrual cycle phase** __pre __pms __have period

Today I physically feel:

_____

_____

*Today I mentally feel:*_____

_____

Any unusual activity or events: _____

_____

Food & Hydration:_____

_____

_____

Medical appointments, procedures or notes: _____

_____

DATE_____

Blood Pressure   sitting ____/____   standing ____/____   Pulse _____BPM

Blood Sugar _____   **Menstrual cycle phase**   __pre   __pms   __have period

Today I physically feel:

_____

_____

*Today I mentally feel:*_____

_____

Any unusual activity or events: _____

_____

Food & Hydration:_____

_____

_____

_____

Medical appointments, procedures or notes: _____

_____

DATE_____

Blood Pressure   sitting ____/____   standing ____/____   Pulse _____BPM

Blood Sugar _____   **Menstrual cycle phase** __pre __pms __have period

Today I physically feel:

_____

_____

*Today I mentally feel:*_____

_____

Any unusual activity or events: _____

_____

Food & Hydration:_____

_____

_____

_____

Medical appointments, procedures or notes: _____

_____

DATE_____

Blood Pressure sitting ____/____   standing ____/____   Pulse _____BPM

Blood Sugar _____   **Menstrual cycle phase** __pre __pms __have period

Today I physically feel:

_____

_____

*Today I mentally feel:*_____

_____

Any unusual activity or events: _____

_____

Food & Hydration:_____

_____

_____

_____

Medical appointments, procedures or notes: _____

_____

DATE_____

Blood Pressure   sitting ____/____   standing ____/____   Pulse _____BPM

Blood Sugar _____   **Menstrual cycle phase** __pre __pms __have period

Today I physically feel:

_____

_____

*Today I mentally feel:*_____

_____

Any unusual activity or events: _____

_____

Food & Hydration:_____

_____

_____

_____

Medical appointments, procedures or notes: _____

_____

DATE_____

Blood Pressure   sitting ____/____   standing ____/____   Pulse _____BPM

Blood Sugar _____   **Menstrual cycle phase** __pre __pms __have period

Today I physically feel:

_____

_____

*Today I mentally feel:*_____

_____

Any unusual activity or events: _____

_____

Food & Hydration:_____

_____

_____

Medical appointments, procedures or notes: _____

_____

DATE_____

Blood Pressure   sitting ____/____   standing ____/____   Pulse _____BPM

Blood Sugar _____   **Menstrual cycle phase**   __pre   __pms   __have period

Today I physically feel:

_____

_____

*Today I mentally feel:*_____

_____

Any unusual activity or events: _____

_____

Food & Hydration:_____

_____

_____

Medical appointments, procedures or notes: _____

_____

DATE_____

Blood Pressure   sitting ____/____   standing ____/____   Pulse _____BPM

Blood Sugar _____   **Menstrual cycle phase** __pre __pms __have period

Today I physically feel:

_____

_____

*Today I mentally feel:*_____

_____

Any unusual activity or events: _____

_____

Food & Hydration:_____

_____

_____

_____

Medical appointments, procedures or notes: _____

_____

DATE_____

Blood Pressure   sitting ____/____   standing ____/____   Pulse _____BPM

Blood Sugar _____   **Menstrual cycle phase**   __pre   __pms   __have period

Today I physically feel:

_____

_____

*Today I mentally feel:*_____

_____

Any unusual activity or events: _____

_____

Food & Hydration:_____

_____

_____

_____

Medical appointments, procedures or notes: _____

_____

DATE_____

Blood Pressure   sitting ____/____   standing ____/____   Pulse _____BPM

Blood Sugar _____   **Menstrual cycle phase** __pre __pms __have period

Today I physically feel:

_____

_____

*Today I mentally feel:*_____

_____

Any unusual activity or events: _____

_____

Food & Hydration:_____

_____

_____

_____

Medical appointments, procedures or notes: _____

_____

DATE_____

Blood Pressure sitting ____/____ standing ____/____ Pulse _____BPM

Blood Sugar _____ **Menstrual cycle phase** __pre __pms __have period

Today I physically feel:

_____

_____

*Today I mentally feel:*_____

_____

Any unusual activity or events: _____

_____

Food & Hydration:_____

_____

_____

_____

Medical appointments, procedures or notes: _____

_____

DATE_____

Blood Pressure   sitting ____/____   standing ____/____   Pulse _____BPM

Blood Sugar _____   **Menstrual cycle phase** __pre __pms __have period

Today I physically feel:

_____

_____

*Today I mentally feel:*_____

_____

Any unusual activity or events: _____

_____

Food & Hydration:_____

_____

_____

Medical appointments, procedures or notes: _____

_____

DATE_____

Blood Pressure sitting ____/____   standing ____/____   Pulse _____BPM

Blood Sugar _____   **Menstrual cycle phase** __pre __pms __have period

Today I physically feel:

_____

_____

*Today I mentally feel:*_____

_____

Any unusual activity or events: _____

_____

*Food & Hydration:*_____

_____

_____

_____

Medical appointments, procedures or notes: _____

_____

DATE_____

Blood Pressure   sitting ____/____   standing ____/____   Pulse _____BPM

Blood Sugar _____   **Menstrual cycle phase** __pre __pms __have period

Today I physically feel:

_____

_____

*Today I mentally feel:*_____

_____

Any unusual activity or events: _____

_____

Food & Hydration:_____

_____

_____

_____

Medical appointments, procedures or notes: _____

_____

DATE_____

Blood Pressure sitting ____/____ standing ____/____ Pulse _____BPM

Blood Sugar _____ **Menstrual cycle phase** __pre __pms __have period

Today I physically feel:

_____

_____

*Today I mentally feel:*_____

_____

Any unusual activity or events: _____

_____

Food & Hydration:_____

_____

_____

_____

Medical appointments, procedures or notes: _____

_____

DATE_____

Blood Pressure sitting ____/____ standing ____/____ Pulse _____BPM

Blood Sugar _____ **Menstrual cycle phase** __pre __pms __have period

Today I physically feel:

_____

_____

*Today I mentally feel:*_____

_____

Any unusual activity or events: _____

_____

Food & Hydration:_____

_____

_____

_____

Medical appointments, procedures or notes: _____

_____

DATE_____

Blood Pressure sitting ____/____ standing ____/____ Pulse _____BPM

Blood Sugar _____ **Menstrual cycle phase** __pre __pms __have period

Today I physically feel:

_____

_____

*Today I mentally feel:*_____

_____

Any unusual activity or events: _____

_____

Food & Hydration:_____

_____

_____

Medical appointments, procedures or notes: _____

_____

DATE_____

Blood Pressure sitting ____/____ standing ____/____ Pulse _____BPM

Blood Sugar _____ **Menstrual cycle phase** __pre __pms __have period

Today I physically feel:

_____

_____

*Today I mentally feel:*_____

_____

Any unusual activity or events: _____

_____

Food & Hydration:_____

_____

_____

Medical appointments, procedures or notes: _____

_____

DATE_____

Blood Pressure   sitting ____/____   standing ____/____   Pulse _____BPM

Blood Sugar _____   **Menstrual cycle phase** __pre __pms __have period

Today I physically feel:

_____

_____

*Today I mentally feel:*_____

_____

Any unusual activity or events: _____

_____

Food & Hydration:_____

_____

_____

_____

Medical appointments, procedures or notes: _____

_____

DATE_____

Blood Pressure   sitting ____/____   standing ____/____   Pulse _____BPM

Blood Sugar _____   **Menstrual cycle phase** __pre __pms __have period

Today I physically feel:

_____

_____

*Today I mentally feel:*_____

_____

Any unusual activity or events: _____

_____

Food & Hydration:_____

_____

_____

_____

Medical appointments, procedures or notes: _____

_____

DATE_____

Blood Pressure sitting ____/____ standing ____/____ Pulse _____BPM

Blood Sugar _____ **Menstrual cycle phase** __pre __pms __have period

Today I physically feel:

_____

_____

*Today I mentally feel:*_____

_____

Any unusual activity or events: _____

_____

Food & Hydration:_____

_____

_____

_____

Medical appointments, procedures or notes: _____

_____

DATE_____

Blood Pressure   sitting ____/____   standing ____/____   Pulse _____BPM

Blood Sugar _____   **Menstrual cycle phase** __pre __pms __have period

Today I physically feel:

_____

_____

*Today I mentally feel:*_____

_____

Any unusual activity or events: _____

_____

Food & Hydration:_____

_____

_____

_____

Medical appointments, procedures or notes: _____

_____

DATE_____

Blood Pressure   sitting ____/____   standing ____/____   Pulse _____BPM

Blood Sugar _____   **Menstrual cycle phase**   __pre   __pms   __have period

Today I physically feel:

_____

_____

*Today I mentally feel:*_____

_____

Any unusual activity or events: _____

_____

Food & Hydration:_____

_____

_____

Medical appointments, procedures or notes: _____

_____

DATE_____

Blood Pressure sitting ____/____   standing ____/____   Pulse _____BPM

Blood Sugar _____   **Menstrual cycle phase** ___pre ___pms ___have period

Today I physically feel:

_____

_____

*Today I mentally feel:*_____

_____

Any unusual activity or events: _____

_____

Food & Hydration:_____

_____

_____

_____

Medical appointments, procedures or notes: _____

_____

DATE_____

Blood Pressure   sitting ____/____   standing ____/____   Pulse _____BPM

Blood Sugar _____   **Menstrual cycle phase** __pre __pms __have period

Today I physically feel:

_____

_____

*Today I mentally feel:*_____

_____

Any unusual activity or events: _____

_____

Food & Hydration:_____

_____

_____

_____

Medical appointments, procedures or notes: _____

_____

What I have learned this month

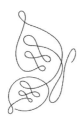

Month & Year

_____

As of the first of the month, I am currently taking the following medications:

Name   Dosage   Frequency

_____   _____   _____

_____   _____   _____

_____   _____   _____

_____   _____   _____

_____   _____   _____

_____   _____   _____

_____   _____   _____

I have the following Dr. appointments and procedures scheduled:

_____

_____

_____

I have the following non-standard activities planned:

_____

_____

_____

DATE_____

Blood Pressure sitting ____/____ standing ____/____ Pulse _____BPM

Blood Sugar _____ **Menstrual cycle phase** __pre __pms __have period

Today I physically feel:

_____

_____

*Today I mentally feel:*_____

_____

Any unusual activity or events: _____

_____

Food & Hydration:_____

_____

_____

_____

Medical appointments, procedures or notes: _____

_____

DATE_____

Blood Pressure   sitting ____/____   standing ____/____   Pulse _____BPM

Blood Sugar _____   **Menstrual cycle phase**   __pre   __pms   __have period

Today I physically feel:

_____

_____

*Today I mentally feel:*_____

_____

Any unusual activity or events: _____

_____

Food & Hydration:_____

_____

_____

_____

Medical appointments, procedures or notes: _____

_____

DATE_____

Blood Pressure sitting ____/____ standing ____/____ Pulse _____BPM

Blood Sugar _____ **Menstrual cycle phase** __pre __pms __have period

Today I physically feel:

_____

_____

*Today I mentally feel:*_____

_____

Any unusual activity or events: _____

_____

Food & Hydration:_____

_____

_____

_____

Medical appointments, procedures or notes: _____

_____

DATE_____

Blood Pressure sitting ____/____ standing ____/____ Pulse _____BPM

Blood Sugar _____ **Menstrual cycle phase** __pre __pms __have period

Today I physically feel:

_____

_____

*Today I mentally feel:*_____

_____

Any unusual activity or events: _____

_____

Food & Hydration:_____

_____

_____

_____

Medical appointments, procedures or notes: _____

_____

DATE_____

Blood Pressure   sitting ____/____   standing ____/____   Pulse _____BPM

Blood Sugar _____   **Menstrual cycle phase** __pre __pms __have period

Today I physically feel:

_____

_____

*Today I mentally feel:*_____

_____

Any unusual activity or events: _____

_____

Food & Hydration:_____

_____

_____

_____

Medical appointments, procedures or notes: _____

_____

DATE_____

Blood Pressure sitting ____/____ standing ____/____ Pulse _____BPM

Blood Sugar _____ **Menstrual cycle phase** __pre __pms __have period

Today I physically feel:

_____

_____

*Today I mentally feel:*_____

_____

Any unusual activity or events: _____

_____

Food & Hydration:_____

_____

_____

Medical appointments, procedures or notes: _____

_____

DATE_____

Blood Pressure   sitting ____/____   standing ____/____   Pulse _____BPM

Blood Sugar _____   **Menstrual cycle phase** __pre __pms __have period

Today I physically feel:

_____

_____

*Today I mentally feel:*_____

_____

Any unusual activity or events: _____

_____

Food & Hydration:_____

_____

_____

_____

Medical appointments, procedures or notes: _____

_____

DATE_____

Blood Pressure sitting ____/____ standing ____/____ Pulse _____BPM

Blood Sugar _____ **Menstrual cycle phase** __pre __pms __have period

Today I physically feel:

_____

_____

*Today I mentally feel:*_____

_____

Any unusual activity or events: _____

_____

Food & Hydration:_____

_____

_____

Medical appointments, procedures or notes: _____

_____

DATE_____

Blood Pressure sitting ____/____   standing ____/____   Pulse _____BPM

Blood Sugar _____   **Menstrual cycle phase** __pre __pms __have period

Today I physically feel:

_____

_____

*Today I mentally feel:*_____

_____

Any unusual activity or events: _____

_____

Food & Hydration:_____

_____

_____

_____

Medical appointments, procedures or notes: _____

_____

DATE_____

Blood Pressure   sitting ____/____   standing ____/____   Pulse _____BPM

Blood Sugar _____   **Menstrual cycle phase**   __pre   __pms   __have period

Today I physically feel:

_____

_____

*Today I mentally feel:*_____

_____

Any unusual activity or events: _____

_____

Food & Hydration:_____

_____

_____

Medical appointments, procedures or notes: _____

_____

DATE_____

Blood Pressure   sitting ____/____   standing ____/____   Pulse _____BPM

Blood Sugar _____   **Menstrual cycle phase** __pre __pms __have period

Today I physically feel:

_____

_____

*Today I mentally feel:*_____

_____

Any unusual activity or events: _____

_____

Food & Hydration:_____

_____

_____

Medical appointments, procedures or notes: _____

_____

DATE_____

Blood Pressure sitting ____/____ standing ____/____ Pulse _____BPM

Blood Sugar _____ **Menstrual cycle phase** __pre __pms __have period

Today I physically feel:

_____

_____

*Today I mentally feel:*_____

_____

Any unusual activity or events: _____

_____

Food & Hydration:_____

_____

_____

Medical appointments, procedures or notes: _____

_____

DATE_____

Blood Pressure   sitting ____/____   standing ____/____   Pulse _____BPM

Blood Sugar _____   **Menstrual cycle phase** __pre __pms __have period

Today I physically feel:

_____

_____

*Today I mentally feel:*_____

_____

Any unusual activity or events: _____

_____

Food & Hydration:_____

_____

_____

_____

Medical appointments, procedures or notes: _____

_____

DATE_____

Blood Pressure   sitting ____/____   standing ____/____   Pulse _____BPM

Blood Sugar _____   **Menstrual cycle phase**   __pre   __pms   __have period

Today I physically feel:

_____

_____

*Today I mentally feel:*_____

_____

Any unusual activity or events: _____

_____

Food & Hydration:_____

_____

_____

_____

Medical appointments, procedures or notes: _____

_____

DATE_____

Blood Pressure sitting ____/____ standing ____/____ Pulse _____BPM

Blood Sugar _____ **Menstrual cycle phase** __pre __pms __have period

Today I physically feel:

_____

_____

*Today I mentally feel:*_____

_____

Any unusual activity or events: _____

_____

Food & Hydration:_____

_____

_____

_____

Medical appointments, procedures or notes: _____

_____

DATE_____

Blood Pressure sitting ____/____   standing ____/____   Pulse _____BPM

Blood Sugar _____   **Menstrual cycle phase** __pre __pms __have period

Today I physically feel:

_____

_____

*Today I mentally feel:*_____

_____

Any unusual activity or events: _____

_____

*Food & Hydration:*_____

_____

_____

_____

Medical appointments, procedures or notes: _____

_____

DATE_____

Blood Pressure   sitting ____/____   standing ____/____   Pulse _____BPM

Blood Sugar _____   **Menstrual cycle phase** __pre __pms __have period

Today I physically feel:

_____

_____

*Today I mentally feel:*_____

_____

Any unusual activity or events: _____

_____

Food & Hydration:_____

_____

_____

_____

Medical appointments, procedures or notes: _____

_____

DATE_____

Blood Pressure sitting ____/____ standing ____/____ Pulse _____BPM

Blood Sugar _____ **Menstrual cycle phase** __pre __pms __have period

Today I physically feel:

_____

_____

*Today I mentally feel:*_____

_____

Any unusual activity or events: _____

_____

Food & Hydration:_____

_____

_____

Medical appointments, procedures or notes: _____

_____

DATE_____

Blood Pressure sitting ____/____ standing ____/____ Pulse _____BPM

Blood Sugar _____ **Menstrual cycle phase** __pre __pms __have period

Today I physically feel:

_____

_____

*Today I mentally feel:*_____

_____

Any unusual activity or events: _____

_____

Food & Hydration:_____

_____

_____

Medical appointments, procedures or notes: _____

_____

DATE_____

Blood Pressure sitting ____/____ standing ____/____ Pulse _____BPM

Blood Sugar _____ **Menstrual cycle phase** __pre __pms __have period

Today I physically feel:

_____

_____

*Today I mentally feel:*_____

_____

Any unusual activity or events: _____

_____

Food & Hydration:_____

_____

_____

Medical appointments, procedures or notes: _____

_____

DATE_____

Blood Pressure   sitting ____/____   standing ____/____   Pulse _____BPM

Blood Sugar _____   **Menstrual cycle phase**   __pre   __pms   __have period

Today I physically feel:

_____

_____

*Today I mentally feel:*_____

_____

Any unusual activity or events: _____

_____

Food & Hydration:_____

_____

_____

_____

Medical appointments, procedures or notes: _____

_____

DATE_____

Blood Pressure sitting ____/____ standing ____/____ Pulse _____BPM

Blood Sugar _____   **Menstrual cycle phase** __pre __pms __have period

Today I physically feel:

_____

_____

*Today I mentally feel:*_____

_____

Any unusual activity or events: _____

_____

Food & Hydration:_____

_____

_____

Medical appointments, procedures or notes: _____

_____

DATE_____

Blood Pressure sitting ____/____ standing ____/____ Pulse ____BPM

Blood Sugar _____ **Menstrual cycle phase** __pre __pms __have period

Today I physically feel:

_____

_____

*Today I mentally feel:*_____

_____

Any unusual activity or events: _____

_____

Food & Hydration:_____

_____

_____

_____

Medical appointments, procedures or notes: _____

_____

DATE_____

Blood Pressure   sitting ____/____   standing ____/____   Pulse _____BPM

Blood Sugar _____   **Menstrual cycle phase** __pre __pms __have period

Today I physically feel:

_____

_____

*Today I mentally feel:*_____

_____

Any unusual activity or events: _____

_____

Food & Hydration:_____

_____

_____

_____

Medical appointments, procedures or notes: _____

_____

DATE_____

Blood Pressure sitting ____/____ standing ____/____ Pulse _____BPM

Blood Sugar _____ **Menstrual cycle phase** __pre __pms __have period

Today I physically feel:

_____

_____

*Today I mentally feel:*_____

_____

Any unusual activity or events: _____

_____

Food & Hydration:_____

_____

_____

_____

Medical appointments, procedures or notes: _____

_____

DATE_____

Blood Pressure   sitting ____/____   standing ____/____   Pulse _____BPM

Blood Sugar _____   **Menstrual cycle phase** __pre __pms __have period

Today I physically feel:

_____

_____

*Today I mentally feel:*_____

_____

Any unusual activity or events: _____

_____

Food & Hydration:_____

_____

_____

_____

Medical appointments, procedures or notes: _____

_____

DATE_____

Blood Pressure   sitting ____/____   standing ____/____   Pulse _____BPM

Blood Sugar _____   **Menstrual cycle phase** __pre __pms __have period

Today I physically feel:

_____

_____

*Today I mentally feel:*_____

_____

Any unusual activity or events: _____

_____

Food & Hydration:_____

_____

_____

_____

Medical appointments, procedures or notes: _____

_____

DATE_____

Blood Pressure   sitting ____/____   standing ____/____   Pulse _____BPM

Blood Sugar _____   **Menstrual cycle phase** __pre __pms __have period

Today I physically feel:

_____

_____

*Today I mentally feel:*_____

_____

Any unusual activity or events: _____

_____

Food & Hydration:_____

_____

_____

Medical appointments, procedures or notes: _____

_____

DATE_____

Blood Pressure sitting ____/____ standing ____/____ Pulse _____BPM

Blood Sugar _____ **Menstrual cycle phase** __pre __pms __have period

Today I physically feel:

_____

_____

*Today I mentally feel:*_____

_____

Any unusual activity or events: _____

_____

Food & Hydration:_____

_____

_____

_____

Medical appointments, procedures or notes: _____

_____

DATE_____

Blood Pressure sitting ____/____ standing ____/____ Pulse _____BPM

Blood Sugar _____ **Menstrual cycle phase** __pre __pms __have period

Today I physically feel:

_____

_____

*Today I mentally feel:*_____

_____

Any unusual activity or events: _____

_____

Food & Hydration:_____

_____

_____

Medical appointments, procedures or notes: _____

_____

DATE_____

Blood Pressure sitting ____/____ standing ____/____ Pulse _____BPM

Blood Sugar _____ **Menstrual cycle phase** __pre __pms __have period

Today I physically feel:

_____

_____

*Today I mentally feel:*_____

_____

Any unusual activity or events: _____

_____

Food & Hydration:_____

_____

_____

_____

Medical appointments, procedures or notes: _____

_____

What I have learned this month

_____

_____

_____

_____

_____

_____

_____

_____

_____

_____

_____

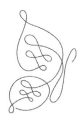

Month & Year

As of the first of the month, I am currently taking the following medications:

Name	Dosage	Frequency

I have the following Dr. appointments and procedures scheduled:

_____

_____

_____

I have the following non-standard activities planned:

_____

_____

_____

DATE_____

Blood Pressure   sitting ____/____   standing ____/____   Pulse _____BPM

Blood Sugar _____   **Menstrual cycle phase** __pre __pms __have period

Today I physically feel:

_____

_____

*Today I mentally feel:*_____

_____

Any unusual activity or events: _____

_____

Food & Hydration:_____

_____

_____

_____

Medical appointments, procedures or notes: _____

_____

DATE_____

Blood Pressure   sitting ____/____   standing ____/____   Pulse _____BPM

Blood Sugar _____   **Menstrual cycle phase** __pre __pms __have period

Today I physically feel:

_____

_____

*Today I mentally feel:*_____

_____

Any unusual activity or events: _____

_____

Food & Hydration:_____

_____

_____

_____

Medical appointments, procedures or notes: _____

_____

DATE_____

Blood Pressure   sitting ____/____   standing ____/____   Pulse _____BPM

Blood Sugar _____   **Menstrual cycle phase** __pre   __pms   __have period

Today I physically feel:

_____

_____

*Today I mentally feel:*_____

_____

Any unusual activity or events: _____

_____

*Food & Hydration:*_____

_____

_____

_____

Medical appointments, procedures or notes: _____

_____

DATE_____

Blood Pressure   sitting ____/____   standing ____/____   Pulse _____BPM

Blood Sugar _____   **Menstrual cycle phase** __pre   __pms   __have period

Today I physically feel:

_____

_____

*Today I mentally feel:*_____

_____

Any unusual activity or events: _____

_____

Food & Hydration:_____

_____

_____

_____

Medical appointments, procedures or notes: _____

_____

DATE_____

Blood Pressure sitting ____/____   standing ____/____   Pulse _____BPM

Blood Sugar _____   **Menstrual cycle phase** __pre __pms __have period

Today I physically feel:

_____

_____

*Today I mentally feel:*_____

_____

Any unusual activity or events: _____

_____

Food & Hydration:_____

_____

_____

Medical appointments, procedures or notes: _____

_____

DATE_____

Blood Pressure   sitting ____/____   standing ____/____   Pulse _____BPM

Blood Sugar _____   **Menstrual cycle phase** __pre __pms __have period

Today I physically feel:

_____

_____

*Today I mentally feel:*_____

_____

Any unusual activity or events: _____

_____

Food & Hydration:_____

_____

_____

_____

Medical appointments, procedures or notes: _____

_____

DATE_____

Blood Pressure   sitting ____/____   standing ____/____   Pulse _____BPM

Blood Sugar _____   **Menstrual cycle phase** __pre __pms __have period

Today I physically feel:

_____

_____

*Today I mentally feel:*_____

_____

Any unusual activity or events: _____

_____

Food & Hydration:_____

_____

_____

_____

Medical appointments, procedures or notes: _____

_____

DATE_____

Blood Pressure   sitting ____/____   standing ____/____   Pulse _____BPM

Blood Sugar _____   **Menstrual cycle phase** __pre   __pms   __have period

Today I physically feel:

_____

_____

*Today I mentally feel:*_____

_____

Any unusual activity or events: _____

_____

Food & Hydration:_____

_____

_____

_____

Medical appointments, procedures or notes: _____

_____

DATE_____

Blood Pressure   sitting ____/____   standing ____/____   Pulse _____BPM

Blood Sugar _____   **Menstrual cycle phase**   __pre   __pms   __have period

Today I physically feel:

_____

_____

*Today I mentally feel:*_____

_____

Any unusual activity or events: _____

_____

Food & Hydration:_____

_____

_____

_____

Medical appointments, procedures or notes: _____

_____

DATE_____

Blood Pressure   sitting ____/____   standing ____/____   Pulse _____BPM

Blood Sugar _____   **Menstrual cycle phase** __pre __pms __have period

Today I physically feel:

_____

_____

*Today I mentally feel:*_____

_____

Any unusual activity or events: _____

_____

Food & Hydration:_____

_____

_____

_____

Medical appointments, procedures or notes: _____

_____

DATE_____

Blood Pressure sitting ____/____ standing ____/____ Pulse _____BPM

Blood Sugar _____   **Menstrual cycle phase** __pre __pms __have period

Today I physically feel:

_____

_____

*Today I mentally feel:*_____

_____

Any unusual activity or events: _____

_____

Food & Hydration:_____

_____

_____

Medical appointments, procedures or notes: _____

_____

DATE_____

Blood Pressure sitting ____/____ standing ____/____ Pulse _____BPM

Blood Sugar _____ **Menstrual cycle phase** __pre __pms __have period

Today I physically feel:

_____

_____

*Today I mentally feel:*_____

_____

Any unusual activity or events: _____

_____

Food & Hydration:_____

_____

_____

_____

Medical appointments, procedures or notes: _____

_____

DATE_____

Blood Pressure sitting ____/____ standing ____/____ Pulse _____BPM

Blood Sugar _____ **Menstrual cycle phase** __pre __pms __have period

Today I physically feel:

_____

_____

*Today I mentally feel:*_____

_____

Any unusual activity or events: _____

_____

Food & Hydration:_____

_____

_____

Medical appointments, procedures or notes: _____

_____

DATE_____

Blood Pressure   sitting ____/____   standing ____/____   Pulse _____BPM

Blood Sugar _____   **Menstrual cycle phase** __pre __pms __have period

Today I physically feel:

_____

_____

*Today I mentally feel:*_____

_____

Any unusual activity or events: _____

_____

Food & Hydration:_____

_____

_____

_____

Medical appointments, procedures or notes: _____

_____

DATE_____

Blood Pressure sitting ____/____   standing ____/____   Pulse _____BPM

Blood Sugar _____   **Menstrual cycle phase** __pre __pms __have period

Today I physically feel:

_____

_____

*Today I mentally feel:*_____

_____

Any unusual activity or events: _____

_____

Food & Hydration:_____

_____

_____

_____

Medical appointments, procedures or notes: _____

_____

DATE_____

Blood Pressure sitting ____/____ standing ____/____ Pulse _____BPM

Blood Sugar _____ **Menstrual cycle phase** __pre __pms __have period

Today I physically feel:

_____

_____

*Today I mentally feel:*_____

_____

Any unusual activity or events: _____

_____

Food & Hydration:_____

_____

_____

Medical appointments, procedures or notes: _____

_____

DATE_____

Blood Pressure sitting ____/____ standing ____/____ Pulse _____BPM

Blood Sugar _____ **Menstrual cycle phase** __pre __pms __have period

Today I physically feel:

_____

_____

*Today I mentally feel:*_____

_____

Any unusual activity or events: _____

_____

Food & Hydration:_____

_____

_____

_____

Medical appointments, procedures or notes: _____

_____

DATE_____

Blood Pressure   sitting ____/____   standing ____/____   Pulse _____BPM

Blood Sugar _____   **Menstrual cycle phase** __pre __pms __have period

Today I physically feel:

_____

_____

*Today I mentally feel:*_____

_____

Any unusual activity or events: _____

_____

Food & Hydration:_____

_____

_____

_____

Medical appointments, procedures or notes: _____

_____

DATE_____

Blood Pressure sitting ____/____   standing ____/____   Pulse _____BPM

Blood Sugar _____   **Menstrual cycle phase** __pre __pms __have period

Today I physically feel:

_____

_____

*Today I mentally feel:*_____

_____

Any unusual activity or events: _____

_____

Food & Hydration:_____

_____

_____

_____

Medical appointments, procedures or notes: _____

_____

DATE_____

Blood Pressure sitting ____/____   standing ____/____   Pulse _____BPM

Blood Sugar _____   **Menstrual cycle phase** __pre __pms __have period

Today I physically feel:

_____

_____

*Today I mentally feel:*_____

_____

Any unusual activity or events: _____

_____

Food & Hydration:_____

_____

_____

_____

Medical appointments, procedures or notes: _____

_____

DATE_____

Blood Pressure sitting ____/____ standing ____/____ Pulse _____BPM

Blood Sugar _____ **Menstrual cycle phase** __pre __pms __have period

Today I physically feel:

_____

_____

*Today I mentally feel:*_____

_____

Any unusual activity or events: _____

_____

Food & Hydration:_____

_____

_____

_____

Medical appointments, procedures or notes: _____

_____

DATE_____

Blood Pressure   sitting ____/____   standing ____/____   Pulse _____BPM

Blood Sugar _____   **Menstrual cycle phase** __pre   __pms   __have period

Today I physically feel:

_____

_____

*Today I mentally feel:*_____

_____

Any unusual activity or events: _____

_____

Food & Hydration:_____

_____

_____

_____

Medical appointments, procedures or notes: _____

_____

DATE_____

Blood Pressure   sitting ____/____   standing ____/____   Pulse _____BPM

Blood Sugar _____   **Menstrual cycle phase**   __pre   __pms   __have period

Today I physically feel:

_____

_____

*Today I mentally feel:*_____

_____

Any unusual activity or events: _____

_____

*Food & Hydration:*_____

_____

_____

_____

Medical appointments, procedures or notes: _____

_____

DATE_____

Blood Pressure sitting ____/____   standing ____/____   Pulse _____BPM

Blood Sugar _____   **Menstrual cycle phase** __pre __pms __have period

Today I physically feel:

_____

_____

*Today I mentally feel:*_____

_____

Any unusual activity or events: _____

_____

Food & Hydration:_____

_____

_____

_____

Medical appointments, procedures or notes: _____

_____

DATE_____

Blood Pressure sitting ____/____ standing ____/____ Pulse _____BPM

Blood Sugar _____ **Menstrual cycle phase** __pre __pms __have period

Today I physically feel:

_____

_____

*Today I mentally feel:*_____

_____

Any unusual activity or events: _____

_____

Food & Hydration:_____

_____

_____

_____

Medical appointments, procedures or notes: _____

_____

DATE_____

Blood Pressure   sitting ____/____   standing ____/____   Pulse _____BPM

Blood Sugar _____   **Menstrual cycle phase** __pre __pms __have period

Today I physically feel:

_____

_____

*Today I mentally feel:*_____

_____

Any unusual activity or events: _____

_____

Food & Hydration:_____

_____

_____

_____

Medical appointments, procedures or notes: _____

_____

DATE_____

Blood Pressure sitting ____/____   standing ____/____   Pulse _____BPM

Blood Sugar _____   **Menstrual cycle phase** __pre __pms __have period

Today I physically feel:

_____

_____

*Today I mentally feel:*_____

_____

Any unusual activity or events: _____

_____

Food & Hydration:_____

_____

_____

Medical appointments, procedures or notes: _____

_____

DATE_____

Blood Pressure   sitting ____/____   standing ____/____   Pulse _____BPM

Blood Sugar _____   **Menstrual cycle phase** __pre   __pms   __have period

Today I physically feel:

_____

_____

*Today I mentally feel:*_____

_____

Any unusual activity or events: _____

_____

Food & Hydration:_____

_____

_____

_____

Medical appointments, procedures or notes: _____

_____

DATE_____

Blood Pressure   sitting ____/____   standing ____/____   Pulse _____BPM

Blood Sugar _____   **Menstrual cycle phase** __pre   __pms   __have period

Today I physically feel:

_____

_____

*Today I mentally feel:*_____

_____

Any unusual activity or events: _____

_____

Food & Hydration:_____

_____

_____

_____

Medical appointments, procedures or notes: _____

_____

DATE_____

Blood Pressure sitting ____/____   standing ____/____   Pulse _____BPM

Blood Sugar _____   **Menstrual cycle phase** __pre __pms __have period

Today I physically feel:

_____

_____

*Today I mentally feel:*_____

_____

Any unusual activity or events: _____

_____

Food & Hydration:_____

_____

_____

_____

Medical appointments, procedures or notes: _____

_____

DATE_____

Blood Pressure sitting ____/____   standing ____/____   Pulse _____BPM

Blood Sugar _____   **Menstrual cycle phase** __pre __pms __have period

Today I physically feel:

_____

_____

*Today I mentally feel:*_____

_____

Any unusual activity or events: _____

_____

Food & Hydration:_____

_____

_____

_____

Medical appointments, procedures or notes: _____

_____

What I have learned this month

_____

_____

_____

_____

_____

_____

_____

_____

_____

_____

_____

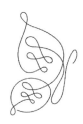

Month & Year

As of the first of the month, I am currently taking the following medications:

Name	Dosage	Frequency
_____	_____	_____
_____	_____	_____
_____	_____	_____
_____	_____	_____
_____	_____	_____
_____	_____	_____
_____	_____	_____

I have the following Dr. appointments and procedures scheduled:

_____

_____

_____

I have the following non-standard activities planned:

_____

_____

_____

DATE_____

Blood Pressure sitting ____/____ standing ____/____ Pulse _____BPM

Blood Sugar _____ **Menstrual cycle phase** __pre __pms __have period

Today I physically feel:

_____

_____

*Today I mentally feel:*_____

_____

Any unusual activity or events: _____

_____

Food & Hydration:_____

_____

_____

Medical appointments, procedures or notes: _____

_____

DATE_____

Blood Pressure sitting ____/____   standing ____/____   Pulse _____BPM

Blood Sugar _____   **Menstrual cycle phase** __pre __pms __have period

Today I physically feel:

_____

_____

*Today I mentally feel:*_____

_____

Any unusual activity or events: _____

_____

Food & Hydration:_____

_____

_____

_____

Medical appointments, procedures or notes: _____

_____

DATE_____

Blood Pressure   sitting ____/____   standing ____/____   Pulse _____BPM

Blood Sugar _____   **Menstrual cycle phase** __pre __pms __have period

Today I physically feel:

_____

_____

*Today I mentally feel:*_____

_____

Any unusual activity or events: _____

_____

Food & Hydration:_____

_____

_____

_____

Medical appointments, procedures or notes: _____

_____

DATE_____

Blood Pressure   sitting ___/___   standing ___/___   Pulse _____BPM

Blood Sugar _____   **Menstrual cycle phase**   __pre   __pms   __have period

Today I physically feel:

_____

_____

*Today I mentally feel:*_____

_____

Any unusual activity or events: _____

_____

Food & Hydration:_____

_____

_____

Medical appointments, procedures or notes: _____

_____

DATE_____

Blood Pressure sitting ____/____   standing ____/____   Pulse _____BPM

Blood Sugar _____   **Menstrual cycle phase** __pre __pms __have period

Today I physically feel:

_____

_____

*Today I mentally feel:*_____

_____

Any unusual activity or events: _____

_____

Food & Hydration:_____

_____

_____

_____

Medical appointments, procedures or notes: _____

_____

DATE_____

Blood Pressure sitting ____/____ standing ____/____ Pulse _____BPM

Blood Sugar _____ **Menstrual cycle phase** __pre __pms __have period

Today I physically feel:

_____

_____

*Today I mentally feel:*_____

_____

Any unusual activity or events: _____

_____

Food & Hydration:_____

_____

_____

Medical appointments, procedures or notes: _____

_____

DATE_____

Blood Pressure   sitting ____/____   standing ____/____   Pulse _____BPM

Blood Sugar _____   **Menstrual cycle phase** __pre __pms __have period

Today I physically feel:

_____

_____

*Today I mentally feel:*_____

_____

Any unusual activity or events: _____

_____

Food & Hydration:_____

_____

_____

_____

Medical appointments, procedures or notes: _____

_____

DATE_____

Blood Pressure sitting ____/____ standing ____/____ Pulse _____BPM

Blood Sugar _____ **Menstrual cycle phase** __pre __pms __have period

Today I physically feel:

_____

_____

*Today I mentally feel:*_____

_____

Any unusual activity or events: _____

_____

Food & Hydration:_____

_____

_____

Medical appointments, procedures or notes: _____

_____

DATE_____

Blood Pressure sitting ____/____ standing ____/____ Pulse _____BPM

Blood Sugar _____ **Menstrual cycle phase** __pre __pms __have period

Today I physically feel:

_____

_____

*Today I mentally feel:*_____

_____

Any unusual activity or events: _____

_____

Food & Hydration:_____

_____

_____

_____

Medical appointments, procedures or notes: _____

_____

DATE_____

Blood Pressure sitting ____/____ standing ____/____ Pulse _____BPM

Blood Sugar _____ **Menstrual cycle phase** __pre __pms __have period

Today I physically feel:

_____

_____

*Today I mentally feel:*_____

_____

Any unusual activity or events: _____

_____

Food & Hydration:_____

_____

_____

Medical appointments, procedures or notes: _____

_____

DATE_____

Blood Pressure sitting ____/____ standing ____/____ Pulse _____BPM

Blood Sugar _____ **Menstrual cycle phase** __pre __pms __have period

Today I physically feel:

_____

_____

*Today I mentally feel:*_____

_____

Any unusual activity or events: _____

_____

Food & Hydration:_____

_____

_____

_____

Medical appointments, procedures or notes: _____

_____

DATE_____

Blood Pressure   sitting ____/____   standing ____/____   Pulse _____BPM

Blood Sugar _____   **Menstrual cycle phase** __pre __pms __have period

Today I physically feel:

_____

_____

*Today I mentally feel:*_____

_____

Any unusual activity or events: _____

_____

Food & Hydration:_____

_____

_____

_____

Medical appointments, procedures or notes: _____

_____

DATE_____

Blood Pressure   sitting ____/____   standing ____/____   Pulse _____BPM

Blood Sugar _____   **Menstrual cycle phase** __pre   __pms   __have period

Today I physically feel:

_____

_____

*Today I mentally feel:*_____

_____

Any unusual activity or events: _____

_____

Food & Hydration:_____

_____

_____

_____

Medical appointments, procedures or notes: _____

_____

DATE_____

Blood Pressure sitting ____/____ standing ____/____ Pulse _____BPM

Blood Sugar _____ **Menstrual cycle phase** __pre __pms __have period

Today I physically feel:

_____

_____

*Today I mentally feel:*_____

_____

Any unusual activity or events: _____

_____

*Food & Hydration:*_____

_____

_____

Medical appointments, procedures or notes: _____

_____

DATE_____

Blood Pressure   sitting ____/____   standing ____/____   Pulse _____BPM

Blood Sugar _____   **Menstrual cycle phase** __pre __pms __have period

Today I physically feel:

_____

_____

*Today I mentally feel:*_____

_____

Any unusual activity or events: _____

_____

Food & Hydration:_____

_____

_____

Medical appointments, procedures or notes: _____

_____

DATE_____

Blood Pressure   sitting ____/____   standing ____/____   Pulse _____BPM

Blood Sugar _____   **Menstrual cycle phase** __pre __pms __have period

Today I physically feel:

_____

_____

*Today I mentally feel:*_____

_____

Any unusual activity or events: _____

_____

Food & Hydration:_____

_____

_____

Medical appointments, procedures or notes: _____

_____

DATE_____

Blood Pressure sitting ____/____   standing ____/____   Pulse _____BPM

Blood Sugar _____   **Menstrual cycle phase** __pre __pms __have period

Today I physically feel:

_____

_____

*Today I mentally feel:*_____

_____

Any unusual activity or events: _____

_____

Food & Hydration:_____

_____

_____

_____

Medical appointments, procedures or notes: _____

_____

DATE_____

Blood Pressure   sitting ____/____   standing ____/____   Pulse _____BPM

Blood Sugar _____   **Menstrual cycle phase** __pre __pms __have period

Today I physically feel:

_____

_____

*Today I mentally feel:*_____

_____

Any unusual activity or events: _____

_____

Food & Hydration:_____

_____

_____

Medical appointments, procedures or notes: _____

_____

DATE_____

Blood Pressure sitting ____/____ standing ____/____ Pulse _____BPM

Blood Sugar _____ **Menstrual cycle phase** __pre __pms __have period

Today I physically feel:

_____

_____

*Today I mentally feel:*_____

_____

Any unusual activity or events: _____

_____

Food & Hydration:_____

_____

_____

_____

Medical appointments, procedures or notes: _____

_____

DATE_____

Blood Pressure sitting ____/____ standing ____/____ Pulse _____BPM

Blood Sugar _____ **Menstrual cycle phase** __pre __pms __have period

Today I physically feel:

_____

_____

*Today I mentally feel:*_____

_____

Any unusual activity or events: _____

_____

Food & Hydration:_____

_____

_____

Medical appointments, procedures or notes: _____

_____

DATE_____

Blood Pressure   sitting ____/____   standing ____/____   Pulse _____BPM

Blood Sugar _____   **Menstrual cycle phase** __pre __pms __have period

Today I physically feel:

_____

_____

*Today I mentally feel:*_____

_____

Any unusual activity or events: _____

_____

Food & Hydration:_____

_____

_____

_____

Medical appointments, procedures or notes: _____

_____

DATE_____

Blood Pressure sitting ____/____   standing ____/____   Pulse _____BPM

Blood Sugar _____   **Menstrual cycle phase** __pre __pms __have period

Today I physically feel:

_____

_____

*Today I mentally feel:*_____

_____

Any unusual activity or events: _____

_____

Food & Hydration:_____

_____

_____

Medical appointments, procedures or notes: _____

_____

DATE_____

Blood Pressure   sitting ____/____   standing ____/____   Pulse _____BPM

Blood Sugar _____   **Menstrual cycle phase** __pre __pms __have period

Today I physically feel:

_____

_____

*Today I mentally feel:*_____

_____

Any unusual activity or events: _____

_____

Food & Hydration:_____

_____

_____

Medical appointments, procedures or notes: _____

_____

DATE_____

Blood Pressure sitting ____/____ standing ____/____ Pulse _____BPM

Blood Sugar _____ **Menstrual cycle phase** __pre __pms __have period

Today I physically feel:

_____

_____

*Today I mentally feel:*_____

_____

Any unusual activity or events: _____

_____

Food & Hydration:_____

_____

_____

Medical appointments, procedures or notes: _____

_____

DATE_____

Blood Pressure sitting ____/____   standing ____/____   Pulse _____BPM

Blood Sugar _____   **Menstrual cycle phase** __pre __pms __have period

Today I physically feel:

_____

_____

*Today I mentally feel:*_____

_____

Any unusual activity or events: _____

_____

Food & Hydration:_____

_____

_____

Medical appointments, procedures or notes: _____

_____

DATE_____

Blood Pressure   sitting ____/____   standing ____/____   Pulse _____BPM

Blood Sugar _____   **Menstrual cycle phase**   __pre   __pms   __have period

Today I physically feel:

_____

_____

*Today I mentally feel:*_____

_____

Any unusual activity or events: _____

_____

Food & Hydration:_____

_____

_____

Medical appointments, procedures or notes: _____

_____

DATE_____

Blood Pressure sitting ____/____   standing ____/____   Pulse _____BPM

Blood Sugar _____   **Menstrual cycle phase** __pre __pms __have period

Today I physically feel:

_____

_____

*Today I mentally feel:*_____

_____

Any unusual activity or events: _____

_____

Food & Hydration:_____

_____

_____

_____

Medical appointments, procedures or notes: _____

_____

DATE_____

Blood Pressure sitting _____/_____ standing _____/_____ Pulse _____BPM

Blood Sugar _____ **Menstrual cycle phase** __pre __pms __have period

Today I physically feel:

_____

_____

*Today I mentally feel:*_____

_____

Any unusual activity or events: _____

_____

Food & Hydration:_____

_____

_____

_____

Medical appointments, procedures or notes: _____

_____

DATE_____

Blood Pressure sitting ____/____ standing ____/____ Pulse _____BPM

Blood Sugar _____ **Menstrual cycle phase** __pre __pms __have period

Today I physically feel:

_____

_____

*Today I mentally feel:*_____

_____

Any unusual activity or events: _____

_____

Food & Hydration:_____

_____

_____

Medical appointments, procedures or notes: _____

_____

DATE_____

Blood Pressure sitting ____/____ standing ____/____ Pulse _____BPM

Blood Sugar _____ **Menstrual cycle phase** __pre __pms __have period

Today I physically feel:

_____

_____

*Today I mentally feel:*_____

_____

Any unusual activity or events: _____

_____

Food & Hydration:_____

_____

_____

_____

Medical appointments, procedures or notes: _____

_____

DATE_____

Blood Pressure sitting ____/____   standing ____/____   Pulse _____BPM

Blood Sugar _____   **Menstrual cycle phase** __pre __pms __have period

Today I physically feel:

_____

_____

*Today I mentally feel:*_____

_____

Any unusual activity or events: _____

_____

Food & Hydration:_____

_____

_____

_____

Medical appointments, procedures or notes: _____

_____

What I have learned this month

_____

_____

_____

_____

_____

_____

_____

_____

_____

_____

_____

_____

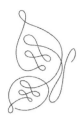

Month & Year

As of the first of the month, I am currently taking the following medications:

Name   Dosage   Frequency

_____   _____   _____

_____   _____   _____

_____   _____   _____

_____   _____   _____

_____   _____   _____

_____   _____   _____

_____   _____   _____

I have the following Dr. appointments and procedures scheduled:

_____

_____

_____

I have the following non-standard activities planned:

_____

_____

_____

DATE_____

Blood Pressure sitting ____/____ standing ____/____ Pulse _____BPM

Blood Sugar _____ **Menstrual cycle phase** __pre __pms __have period

Today I physically feel:

_____

_____

*Today I mentally feel:*_____

_____

Any unusual activity or events: _____

_____

Food & Hydration:_____

_____

_____

Medical appointments, procedures or notes: _____

_____

DATE_____

Blood Pressure sitting ____/____   standing ____/____   Pulse _____BPM

Blood Sugar _____   **Menstrual cycle phase** __pre __pms __have period

Today I physically feel:

_____

_____

*Today I mentally feel:*_____

_____

Any unusual activity or events: _____

_____

Food & Hydration:_____

_____

_____

_____

Medical appointments, procedures or notes: _____

_____

DATE_____

Blood Pressure   sitting ____/____   standing ____/____   Pulse _____BPM

Blood Sugar _____   **Menstrual cycle phase**   __pre   __pms   __have period

Today I physically feel:

_____

_____

*Today I mentally feel:*_____

_____

Any unusual activity or events: _____

_____

Food & Hydration:_____

_____

_____

_____

Medical appointments, procedures or notes: _____

_____

DATE_____

Blood Pressure   sitting ____/____   standing ____/____   Pulse _____BPM

Blood Sugar _____   **Menstrual cycle phase** __pre __pms __have period

Today I physically feel:

_____

_____

*Today I mentally feel:*_____

_____

Any unusual activity or events: _____

_____

Food & Hydration:_____

_____

_____

Medical appointments, procedures or notes: _____

_____

DATE_____

Blood Pressure sitting ____/____ standing ____/____ Pulse _____BPM

Blood Sugar _____ **Menstrual cycle phase** __pre __pms __have period

Today I physically feel:

_____

_____

*Today I mentally feel:*_____

_____

Any unusual activity or events: _____

_____

Food & Hydration:_____

_____

_____

_____

Medical appointments, procedures or notes: _____

_____

DATE_____

Blood Pressure sitting ____/____ standing ____/____ Pulse _____BPM

Blood Sugar _____ **Menstrual cycle phase** __pre __pms __have period

Today I physically feel:

_____

_____

*Today I mentally feel:*_____

_____

Any unusual activity or events: _____

_____

Food & Hydration:_____

_____

_____

_____

Medical appointments, procedures or notes: _____

_____

DATE_____

Blood Pressure sitting ____/____ standing ____/____ Pulse _____BPM

Blood Sugar _____ **Menstrual cycle phase** __pre __pms __have period

Today I physically feel:

_____

_____

*Today I mentally feel:*_____

_____

Any unusual activity or events: _____

_____

Food & Hydration:_____

_____

_____

_____

Medical appointments, procedures or notes: _____

_____

DATE_____

Blood Pressure sitting ____/____ standing ____/____ Pulse _____BPM

Blood Sugar _____ **Menstrual cycle phase** __pre __pms __have period

Today I physically feel:

_____

_____

*Today I mentally feel:*_____

_____

Any unusual activity or events: _____

_____

Food & Hydration:_____

_____

_____

_____

Medical appointments, procedures or notes: _____

_____

DATE_____

Blood Pressure sitting ____/____ standing ____/____ Pulse _____BPM

Blood Sugar _____ **Menstrual cycle phase** __pre __pms __have period

Today I physically feel:

_____

_____

*Today I mentally feel:*_____

_____

Any unusual activity or events: _____

_____

*Food & Hydration:*_____

_____

_____

_____

Medical appointments, procedures or notes: _____

_____

DATE_____

Blood Pressure sitting ____/____ standing ____/____ Pulse _____BPM

Blood Sugar _____ **Menstrual cycle phase** __pre __pms __have period

Today I physically feel:

_____

_____

*Today I mentally feel:*_____

_____

Any unusual activity or events: _____

_____

Food & Hydration:_____

_____

_____

_____

Medical appointments, procedures or notes: _____

_____

DATE_____

Blood Pressure sitting ____/____   standing ____/____   Pulse _____BPM

Blood Sugar _____   **Menstrual cycle phase** __pre   __pms   __have period

Today I physically feel:

_____

_____

*Today I mentally feel:*_____

_____

Any unusual activity or events: _____

_____

Food & Hydration:_____

_____

_____

_____

Medical appointments, procedures or notes: _____

_____

DATE_____

Blood Pressure sitting ____/____ standing ____/____ Pulse _____BPM

Blood Sugar _____ **Menstrual cycle phase** __pre __pms __have period

Today I physically feel:

_____

_____

*Today I mentally feel:*_____

_____

Any unusual activity or events: _____

_____

Food & Hydration:_____

_____

_____

_____

Medical appointments, procedures or notes: _____

_____

DATE_____

Blood Pressure sitting ____/____   standing ____/____   Pulse _____BPM

Blood Sugar _____   **Menstrual cycle phase** __pre __pms __have period

Today I physically feel:

_____

_____

*Today I mentally feel:*_____

_____

Any unusual activity or events: _____

_____

Food & Hydration:_____

_____

_____

_____

Medical appointments, procedures or notes: _____

_____

DATE_____

Blood Pressure   sitting ____/____   standing ____/____   Pulse _____BPM

Blood Sugar _____   **Menstrual cycle phase** __pre __pms __have period

Today I physically feel:

_____

_____

*Today I mentally feel:*_____

_____

Any unusual activity or events: _____

_____

Food & Hydration:_____

_____

_____

Medical appointments, procedures or notes: _____

_____

DATE_____

Blood Pressure   sitting ____/____   standing ____/____   Pulse _____BPM

Blood Sugar _____   **Menstrual cycle phase** __pre __pms __have period

Today I physically feel:

_____

_____

*Today I mentally feel:*_____

_____

Any unusual activity or events: _____

_____

*Food & Hydration:*_____

_____

_____

_____

Medical appointments, procedures or notes: _____

_____

DATE_____

Blood Pressure   sitting _____/_____   standing _____/_____   Pulse _____BPM

Blood Sugar _____   **Menstrual cycle phase** __pre   __pms   __have period

Today I physically feel:

_____

_____

*Today I mentally feel:*_____

_____

Any unusual activity or events: _____

_____

Food & Hydration:_____

_____

_____

_____

Medical appointments, procedures or notes: _____

_____

DATE_____

Blood Pressure   sitting ____/____   standing ____/____   Pulse _____BPM

Blood Sugar _____   **Menstrual cycle phase** __pre __pms __have period

Today I physically feel:

_____

_____

*Today I mentally feel:*_____

_____

Any unusual activity or events: _____

_____

Food & Hydration:_____

_____

_____

_____

Medical appointments, procedures or notes: _____

_____

DATE_____

Blood Pressure   sitting ____/____   standing ____/____   Pulse _____BPM

Blood Sugar _____   **Menstrual cycle phase** __pre   __pms   __have period

Today I physically feel:

_____

_____

*Today I mentally feel:*_____

_____

Any unusual activity or events: _____

_____

Food & Hydration:_____

_____

_____

_____

Medical appointments, procedures or notes: _____

_____

DATE_____

Blood Pressure sitting ____/____ standing ____/____ Pulse _____BPM

Blood Sugar _____ **Menstrual cycle phase** __pre __pms __have period

Today I physically feel:

_____

_____

*Today I mentally feel:*_____

_____

Any unusual activity or events: _____

_____

Food & Hydration:_____

_____

_____

_____

Medical appointments, procedures or notes: _____

_____

DATE_____

Blood Pressure   sitting ____/____   standing ____/____   Pulse _____BPM

Blood Sugar _____   **Menstrual cycle phase**   __pre   __pms   __have period

Today I physically feel:

_____

_____

*Today I mentally feel:*_____

_____

Any unusual activity or events: _____

_____

Food & Hydration:_____

_____

_____

Medical appointments, procedures or notes: _____

_____

DATE_____

Blood Pressure sitting ____/____ standing ____/____ Pulse _____BPM

Blood Sugar _____ **Menstrual cycle phase** __pre __pms __have period

Today I physically feel:

_____

_____

*Today I mentally feel:*_____

_____

Any unusual activity or events: _____

_____

Food & Hydration:_____

_____

_____

_____

Medical appointments, procedures or notes: _____

_____

DATE_____

Blood Pressure sitting ____/____ standing ____/____ Pulse _____BPM

Blood Sugar _____ **Menstrual cycle phase** __pre __pms __have period

Today I physically feel:

_____

_____

*Today I mentally feel:*_____

_____

Any unusual activity or events: _____

_____

Food & Hydration:_____

_____

_____

_____

Medical appointments, procedures or notes: _____

_____

DATE_____

Blood Pressure   sitting ____/____   standing ____/____   Pulse _____BPM

Blood Sugar _____   **Menstrual cycle phase**   __pre   __pms   __have period

Today I physically feel:

_____

_____

*Today I mentally feel:*_____

_____

Any unusual activity or events: _____

_____

Food & Hydration:_____

_____

_____

_____

Medical appointments, procedures or notes: _____

_____

DATE_____

Blood Pressure sitting ____/____ standing ____/____ Pulse _____BPM

Blood Sugar _____   **Menstrual cycle phase** __pre __pms __have period

Today I physically feel:

_____

_____

*Today I mentally feel:*_____

_____

Any unusual activity or events: _____

_____

Food & Hydration:_____

_____

_____

Medical appointments, procedures or notes: _____

_____

DATE_____

Blood Pressure sitting ____/____ standing ____/____ Pulse _____BPM

Blood Sugar _____ **Menstrual cycle phase** __pre __pms __have period

Today I physically feel:

_____

_____

*Today I mentally feel:*_____

_____

Any unusual activity or events: _____

_____

Food & Hydration:_____

_____

_____

_____

Medical appointments, procedures or notes: _____

_____

DATE_____

Blood Pressure sitting ____/____   standing ____/____   Pulse _____BPM

Blood Sugar _____   **Menstrual cycle phase** __pre   __pms   __have period

Today I physically feel:

_____

_____

*Today I mentally feel:*_____

_____

Any unusual activity or events: _____

_____

Food & Hydration:_____

_____

_____

Medical appointments, procedures or notes: _____

_____

DATE_____

Blood Pressure sitting ____/____ standing ____/____ Pulse _____BPM

Blood Sugar _____ **Menstrual cycle phase** __pre __pms __have period

Today I physically feel:

_____

_____

*Today I mentally feel:*_____

_____

Any unusual activity or events: _____

_____

Food & Hydration:_____

_____

_____

_____

Medical appointments, procedures or notes: _____

_____

DATE_____

Blood Pressure   sitting ____/____   standing ____/____   Pulse _____BPM

Blood Sugar _____   **Menstrual cycle phase** __pre __pms __have period

Today I physically feel:

_____

_____

*Today I mentally feel:*_____

_____

Any unusual activity or events: _____

_____

Food & Hydration:_____

_____

_____

_____

Medical appointments, procedures or notes: _____

_____

DATE_____

Blood Pressure sitting ____/____ standing ____/____ Pulse _____BPM

Blood Sugar _____ **Menstrual cycle phase** __pre __pms __have period

Today I physically feel:

_____

_____

*Today I mentally feel:*_____

_____

Any unusual activity or events: _____

_____

*Food & Hydration:*_____

_____

_____

_____

Medical appointments, procedures or notes: _____

_____

DATE_____

Blood Pressure sitting ____/____ standing ____/____ Pulse _____BPM

Blood Sugar _____ **Menstrual cycle phase** __pre __pms __have period

Today I physically feel:

_____

_____

*Today I mentally feel:*_____

_____

Any unusual activity or events: _____

_____

Food & Hydration:_____

_____

_____

_____

Medical appointments, procedures or notes: _____

_____

DATE_____

Blood Pressure sitting ____/____ standing ____/____ Pulse _____BPM

Blood Sugar _____ **Menstrual cycle phase** __pre __pms __have period

Today I physically feel:

_____

_____

*Today I mentally feel:*_____

_____

Any unusual activity or events: _____

_____

Food & Hydration:_____

_____

_____

Medical appointments, procedures or notes: _____

_____

What I have learned this month

_____

_____

_____

_____

_____

_____

_____

_____

_____

_____

_____

_____

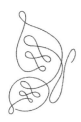

Month & Year

As of the first of the month, I am currently taking the following medications:

Name	Dosage	Frequency

I have the following Dr. appointments and procedures scheduled:

_____

_____

_____

I have the following non-standard activities planned:

_____

_____

_____

DATE_____

Blood Pressure   sitting ____/____   standing ____/____   Pulse _____BPM

Blood Sugar _____   **Menstrual cycle phase** __pre   __pms   __have period

Today I physically feel:

_____

_____

*Today I mentally feel:*_____

_____

Any unusual activity or events: _____

_____

Food & Hydration:_____

_____

_____

_____

Medical appointments, procedures or notes: _____

_____

DATE_____

Blood Pressure   sitting ____/____   standing ____/____   Pulse _____BPM

Blood Sugar _____   **Menstrual cycle phase** __pre __pms __have period

Today I physically feel:

_____

_____

*Today I mentally feel:*_____

_____

Any unusual activity or events: _____

_____

Food & Hydration:_____

_____

_____

_____

Medical appointments, procedures or notes: _____

_____

DATE_____

Blood Pressure sitting ____/____ standing ____/____ Pulse _____BPM

Blood Sugar _____ **Menstrual cycle phase** __pre __pms __have period

Today I physically feel:

_____

_____

*Today I mentally feel:*_____

_____

Any unusual activity or events: _____

_____

Food & Hydration:_____

_____

_____

_____

Medical appointments, procedures or notes: _____

_____

DATE_____

Blood Pressure   sitting ____/____   standing ____/____   Pulse _____BPM

Blood Sugar _____   **Menstrual cycle phase**   __pre   __pms   __have period

Today I physically feel:

_____

_____

*Today I mentally feel:*_____

_____

Any unusual activity or events: _____

_____

Food & Hydration:_____

_____

_____

Medical appointments, procedures or notes: _____

_____

DATE_____

Blood Pressure sitting ____/____   standing ____/____   Pulse _____BPM

Blood Sugar _____   **Menstrual cycle phase** __pre   __pms   __have period

Today I physically feel:

_____

_____

*Today I mentally feel:*_____

_____

Any unusual activity or events: _____

_____

Food & Hydration:_____

_____

_____

_____

Medical appointments, procedures or notes: _____

_____

DATE_____

Blood Pressure sitting ____/____ standing ____/____ Pulse _____BPM

Blood Sugar _____ **Menstrual cycle phase** __pre __pms __have period

Today I physically feel:

_____

_____

*Today I mentally feel:*_____

_____

Any unusual activity or events: _____

_____

Food & Hydration:_____

_____

_____

_____

Medical appointments, procedures or notes: _____

_____

DATE_____

Blood Pressure sitting ____/____   standing ____/____   Pulse _____BPM

Blood Sugar _____   **Menstrual cycle phase** __pre __pms __have period

Today I physically feel:

_____

_____

*Today I mentally feel:*_____

_____

Any unusual activity or events: _____

_____

Food & Hydration:_____

_____

_____

Medical appointments, procedures or notes: _____

_____

DATE_____

Blood Pressure sitting ____/____ standing ____/____ Pulse _____BPM

Blood Sugar _____ **Menstrual cycle phase** __pre __pms __have period

Today I physically feel:

_____

_____

*Today I mentally feel:*_____

_____

Any unusual activity or events: _____

_____

Food & Hydration:_____

_____

_____

_____

Medical appointments, procedures or notes: _____

_____

DATE_____

Blood Pressure sitting ____/____   standing ____/____   Pulse _____BPM

Blood Sugar _____   **Menstrual cycle phase** __pre   __pms   __have period

Today I physically feel:

_____

_____

*Today I mentally feel:*_____

_____

Any unusual activity or events: _____

_____

Food & Hydration:_____

_____

_____

Medical appointments, procedures or notes: _____

_____

DATE_____

Blood Pressure sitting ____/____   standing ____/____   Pulse _____BPM

Blood Sugar _____   **Menstrual cycle phase** __pre __pms __have period

Today I physically feel:

_____

_____

*Today I mentally feel:*_____

_____

Any unusual activity or events: _____

_____

Food & Hydration:_____

_____

_____

Medical appointments, procedures or notes: _____

_____

DATE_____

Blood Pressure sitting ____/____ standing ____/____ Pulse _____BPM

Blood Sugar _____   **Menstrual cycle phase** __pre __pms __have period

Today I physically feel:

_____

_____

*Today I mentally feel:*_____

_____

Any unusual activity or events: _____

_____

Food & Hydration:_____

_____

_____

_____

Medical appointments, procedures or notes: _____

_____

DATE_____

Blood Pressure   sitting ____/____   standing ____/____   Pulse _____BPM

Blood Sugar _____   **Menstrual cycle phase** __pre __pms __have period

Today I physically feel:

_____

_____

*Today I mentally feel:*_____

_____

Any unusual activity or events: _____

_____

Food & Hydration:_____

_____

_____

Medical appointments, procedures or notes: _____

_____

DATE_____

Blood Pressure sitting ____/____ standing ____/____ Pulse _____BPM

Blood Sugar _____ **Menstrual cycle phase** __pre __pms __have period

Today I physically feel:

_____

_____

*Today I mentally feel:*_____

_____

Any unusual activity or events: _____

_____

Food & Hydration:_____

_____

_____

Medical appointments, procedures or notes: _____

_____

DATE_____

Blood Pressure   sitting ____/____   standing ____/____   Pulse _____BPM

Blood Sugar _____   **Menstrual cycle phase** __pre __pms __have period

Today I physically feel:

_____

_____

*Today I mentally feel:*_____

_____

Any unusual activity or events: _____

_____

*Food & Hydration:*_____

_____

_____

_____

Medical appointments, procedures or notes: _____

_____

DATE_____

Blood Pressure sitting ____/____   standing ____/____   Pulse _____BPM

Blood Sugar _____   **Menstrual cycle phase** __pre __pms __have period

Today I physically feel:

_____

_____

*Today I mentally feel:*_____

_____

Any unusual activity or events: _____

_____

Food & Hydration:_____

_____

_____

_____

Medical appointments, procedures or notes: _____

_____

DATE_____

Blood Pressure sitting ____/____   standing ____/____   Pulse _____BPM

Blood Sugar _____   **Menstrual cycle phase** __pre   __pms   __have period

Today I physically feel:

_____

_____

*Today I mentally feel:*_____

_____

Any unusual activity or events: _____

_____

*Food & Hydration:*_____

_____

_____

Medical appointments, procedures or notes: _____

_____

DATE_____

Blood Pressure sitting ____/____   standing ____/____   Pulse _____BPM

Blood Sugar _____   **Menstrual cycle phase** __pre __pms __have period

Today I physically feel:

_____

_____

*Today I mentally feel:*_____

_____

Any unusual activity or events: _____

_____

Food & Hydration:_____

_____

_____

_____

Medical appointments, procedures or notes: _____

_____

DATE_____

Blood Pressure   sitting ___/___   standing ___/___   Pulse ____BPM

Blood Sugar _____   **Menstrual cycle phase**   __pre   __pms   __have period

Today I physically feel:

_____

_____

*Today I mentally feel:*_____

_____

Any unusual activity or events: _____

_____

Food & Hydration:_____

_____

_____

Medical appointments, procedures or notes: _____

_____

DATE_____

Blood Pressure sitting ____/____   standing ____/____   Pulse _____BPM

Blood Sugar _____   **Menstrual cycle phase** __pre __pms __have period

Today I physically feel:

_____

_____

*Today I mentally feel:*_____

_____

Any unusual activity or events: _____

_____

Food & Hydration:_____

_____

_____

Medical appointments, procedures or notes: _____

_____

DATE_____

Blood Pressure   sitting ____/____   standing ____/____   Pulse _____BPM

Blood Sugar _____   **Menstrual cycle phase** __pre   __pms   __have period

Today I physically feel:

_____

_____

*Today I mentally feel:*_____

_____

Any unusual activity or events: _____

_____

Food & Hydration:_____

_____

_____

_____

Medical appointments, procedures or notes: _____

_____

DATE_____

Blood Pressure sitting ____/____   standing ____/____   Pulse _____BPM

Blood Sugar _____   **Menstrual cycle phase** __pre __pms __have period

Today I physically feel:

_____

_____

*Today I mentally feel:*_____

_____

Any unusual activity or events: _____

_____

Food & Hydration:_____

_____

_____

Medical appointments, procedures or notes: _____

_____

DATE_____

Blood Pressure sitting ____/____ standing ____/____ Pulse _____BPM

Blood Sugar _____ **Menstrual cycle phase** __pre __pms __have period

Today I physically feel:

_____

_____

*Today I mentally feel:*_____

_____

Any unusual activity or events: _____

_____

Food & Hydration:_____

_____

_____

Medical appointments, procedures or notes: _____

_____

DATE_____

Blood Pressure   sitting ____/____   standing ____/____   Pulse _____BPM

Blood Sugar _____   **Menstrual cycle phase** __pre __pms __have period

Today I physically feel:

_____

_____

*Today I mentally feel:*_____

_____

Any unusual activity or events: _____

_____

Food & Hydration:_____

_____

_____

Medical appointments, procedures or notes: _____

_____

DATE_____

Blood Pressure sitting ____/____   standing ____/____   Pulse _____BPM

Blood Sugar _____   **Menstrual cycle phase** __pre   __pms   __have period

Today I physically feel:

_____

_____

*Today I mentally feel:*_____

_____

Any unusual activity or events: _____

_____

Food & Hydration:_____

_____

_____

_____

Medical appointments, procedures or notes: _____

_____

DATE_____

Blood Pressure sitting ____/____   standing ____/____   Pulse _____BPM

Blood Sugar _____   **Menstrual cycle phase** __pre   __pms   __have period

Today I physically feel:

_____

_____

*Today I mentally feel:*_____

_____

Any unusual activity or events: _____

_____

Food & Hydration:_____

_____

_____

Medical appointments, procedures or notes: _____

_____

DATE_____

Blood Pressure   sitting ____/____   standing ____/____   Pulse _____BPM

Blood Sugar _____   **Menstrual cycle phase** __pre __pms __have period

Today I physically feel:

_____

_____

*Today I mentally feel:*_____

_____

Any unusual activity or events: _____

_____

Food & Hydration:_____

_____

_____

Medical appointments, procedures or notes: _____

_____

DATE_____

Blood Pressure sitting ____/____   standing ____/____   Pulse _____BPM

Blood Sugar _____   **Menstrual cycle phase** __pre   __pms   __have period

Today I physically feel:

_____

_____

*Today I mentally feel:*_____

_____

Any unusual activity or events: _____

_____

Food & Hydration:_____

_____

_____

Medical appointments, procedures or notes: _____

_____

DATE_____

Blood Pressure sitting ____/____ standing ____/____ Pulse _____BPM

Blood Sugar _____   **Menstrual cycle phase** __pre __pms __have period

Today I physically feel:

_____

_____

*Today I mentally feel:*_____

_____

Any unusual activity or events: _____

_____

Food & Hydration:_____

_____

_____

_____

Medical appointments, procedures or notes: _____

_____

DATE_____

Blood Pressure   sitting ____/____   standing ____/____   Pulse _____BPM

Blood Sugar _____   **Menstrual cycle phase** __pre   __pms   __have period

Today I physically feel:

_____

_____

*Today I mentally feel:*_____

_____

Any unusual activity or events: _____

_____

Food & Hydration:_____

_____

_____

_____

Medical appointments, procedures or notes: _____

_____

DATE_____

Blood Pressure sitting ____/____ standing ____/____ Pulse _____BPM

Blood Sugar _____ **Menstrual cycle phase** __pre __pms __have period

Today I physically feel:

_____

_____

*Today I mentally feel:*_____

_____

Any unusual activity or events: _____

_____

Food & Hydration:_____

_____

_____

Medical appointments, procedures or notes: _____

_____

DATE_____

Blood Pressure sitting ____/____ standing ____/____ Pulse _____BPM

Blood Sugar _____ **Menstrual cycle phase** __pre __pms __have period

Today I physically feel:

_____

_____

*Today I mentally feel:*_____

_____

Any unusual activity or events: _____

_____

Food & Hydration:_____

_____

_____

Medical appointments, procedures or notes: _____

_____

What I have learned this month

_____

_____

_____

_____

_____

_____

_____

_____

_____

_____

_____

_____

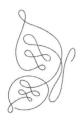

Month & Year

As of the first of the month, I am currently taking the following medications:

Name   Dosage   Frequency

_____   _____   _____

_____   _____   _____

_____   _____   _____

_____   _____   _____

_____   _____   _____

_____   _____   _____

_____   _____   _____

I have the following Dr. appointments and procedures scheduled:

_____

_____

_____

I have the following non-standard activities planned:

_____

_____

_____

DATE_____

Blood Pressure   sitting ____/____   standing ____/____   Pulse _____BPM

Blood Sugar _____   **Menstrual cycle phase** __pre   __pms   __have period

Today I physically feel:

_____

_____

*Today I mentally feel:*_____

_____

Any unusual activity or events: _____

_____

Food & Hydration:_____

_____

_____

_____

Medical appointments, procedures or notes: _____

_____

DATE_____

Blood Pressure sitting ____/____ standing ____/____ Pulse _____BPM

Blood Sugar _____ **Menstrual cycle phase** __pre __pms __have period

Today I physically feel:

_____

_____

*Today I mentally feel:*_____

_____

Any unusual activity or events: _____

_____

Food & Hydration:_____

_____

_____

_____

Medical appointments, procedures or notes: _____

_____

DATE_____

Blood Pressure   sitting ____/____   standing ____/____   Pulse _____BPM

Blood Sugar _____   **Menstrual cycle phase**   __pre   __pms   __have period

Today I physically feel:

_____

_____

*Today I mentally feel:*_____

_____

Any unusual activity or events: _____

_____

Food & Hydration:_____

_____

_____

Medical appointments, procedures or notes: _____

_____

DATE_____

Blood Pressure sitting ____/____ standing ____/____ Pulse _____BPM

Blood Sugar _____ **Menstrual cycle phase** __pre __pms __have period

Today I physically feel:

_____

_____

*Today I mentally feel:*_____

_____

Any unusual activity or events: _____

_____

Food & Hydration:_____

_____

_____

_____

Medical appointments, procedures or notes: _____

_____

DATE_____

Blood Pressure sitting ____/____   standing ____/____   Pulse _____BPM

Blood Sugar _____   **Menstrual cycle phase** __pre __pms __have period

Today I physically feel:

_____

_____

*Today I mentally feel:*_____

_____

Any unusual activity or events: _____

_____

Food & Hydration:_____

_____

_____

Medical appointments, procedures or notes: _____

_____

DATE_____

Blood Pressure sitting ____/____ standing ____/____ Pulse _____BPM

Blood Sugar _____ **Menstrual cycle phase** __pre __pms __have period

Today I physically feel:

_____

_____

*Today I mentally feel:*_____

_____

Any unusual activity or events: _____

_____

Food & Hydration:_____

_____

_____

Medical appointments, procedures or notes: _____

_____

DATE_____

Blood Pressure sitting ____/____   standing ____/____   Pulse _____BPM

Blood Sugar _____   **Menstrual cycle phase** __pre __pms __have period

Today I physically feel:

_____

_____

*Today I mentally feel:*_____

_____

Any unusual activity or events: _____

_____

Food & Hydration:_____

_____

_____

_____

Medical appointments, procedures or notes: _____

_____

DATE_____

Blood Pressure sitting ____/____   standing ____/____   Pulse _____BPM

Blood Sugar _____   **Menstrual cycle phase** __pre __pms __have period

Today I physically feel:

_____

_____

*Today I mentally feel:*_____

_____

Any unusual activity or events: _____

_____

Food & Hydration:_____

_____

_____

Medical appointments, procedures or notes: _____

_____

DATE_____

Blood Pressure   sitting ____/____   standing ____/____   Pulse _____BPM

Blood Sugar _____   **Menstrual cycle phase** __pre __pms __have period

Today I physically feel:

_____

_____

*Today I mentally feel:*_____

_____

Any unusual activity or events: _____

_____

Food & Hydration:_____

_____

_____

_____

Medical appointments, procedures or notes: _____

_____

DATE_____

Blood Pressure   sitting ____/____   standing ____/____   Pulse _____BPM

Blood Sugar _____   **Menstrual cycle phase** __pre __pms __have period

Today I physically feel:

_____

_____

*Today I mentally feel:*_____

_____

Any unusual activity or events: _____

_____

Food & Hydration:_____

_____

_____

Medical appointments, procedures or notes: _____

_____

DATE_____

Blood Pressure   sitting ____/____   standing ____/____   Pulse _____BPM

Blood Sugar _____   **Menstrual cycle phase**   __pre   __pms   __have period

Today I physically feel:

_____

_____

*Today I mentally feel:*_____

_____

Any unusual activity or events: _____

_____

Food & Hydration:_____

_____

_____

_____

Medical appointments, procedures or notes: _____

_____

DATE_____

Blood Pressure sitting ____/____   standing ____/____   Pulse _____BPM

Blood Sugar _____   **Menstrual cycle phase** __pre __pms __have period

Today I physically feel:

_____

_____

*Today I mentally feel:*_____

_____

Any unusual activity or events: _____

_____

Food & Hydration:_____

_____

_____

Medical appointments, procedures or notes: _____

_____

DATE_____

Blood Pressure sitting ____/____   standing ____/____   Pulse _____BPM

Blood Sugar _____   **Menstrual cycle phase** __pre __pms __have period

Today I physically feel:

_____

_____

*Today I mentally feel:*_____

_____

Any unusual activity or events: _____

_____

Food & Hydration:_____

_____

_____

_____

Medical appointments, procedures or notes: _____

_____

DATE_____

Blood Pressure sitting ____/____   standing ____/____   Pulse _____BPM

Blood Sugar _____   **Menstrual cycle phase** __pre __pms __have period

Today I physically feel:

_____

_____

*Today I mentally feel:*_____

_____

Any unusual activity or events: _____

_____

Food & Hydration:_____

_____

_____

Medical appointments, procedures or notes: _____

_____

DATE_____

Blood Pressure sitting ____/____   standing ____/____   Pulse _____BPM

Blood Sugar _____   **Menstrual cycle phase** __pre __pms __have period

Today I physically feel:

_____

_____

*Today I mentally feel:*_____

_____

Any unusual activity or events: _____

_____

Food & Hydration:_____

_____

_____

_____

Medical appointments, procedures or notes: _____

_____

DATE_____

Blood Pressure sitting ____/____ standing ____/____ Pulse _____BPM

Blood Sugar _____ **Menstrual cycle phase** __pre __pms __have period

Today I physically feel:

_____

_____

*Today I mentally feel:*_____

_____

Any unusual activity or events: _____

_____

Food & Hydration:_____

_____

_____

_____

Medical appointments, procedures or notes: _____

_____

DATE_____

Blood Pressure sitting ____/____   standing ____/____   Pulse _____BPM

Blood Sugar _____   **Menstrual cycle phase** __pre __pms __have period

Today I physically feel:

_____

_____

*Today I mentally feel:*_____

_____

Any unusual activity or events: _____

_____

Food & Hydration:_____

_____

_____

_____

Medical appointments, procedures or notes: _____

_____

DATE_____

Blood Pressure   sitting ____/____   standing ____/____   Pulse _____BPM

Blood Sugar _____   **Menstrual cycle phase** __pre __pms __have period

Today I physically feel:

_____

_____

*Today I mentally feel:*_____

_____

Any unusual activity or events: _____

_____

Food & Hydration:_____

_____

_____

_____

Medical appointments, procedures or notes: _____

_____

DATE_____

Blood Pressure sitting ____/____ standing ____/____ Pulse _____BPM

Blood Sugar _____ **Menstrual cycle phase** __pre __pms __have period

Today I physically feel:

_____

_____

*Today I mentally feel:*_____

_____

Any unusual activity or events: _____

_____

Food & Hydration:_____

_____

_____

_____

Medical appointments, procedures or notes: _____

_____

DATE_____

Blood Pressure   sitting ____/____   standing ____/____   Pulse _____BPM

Blood Sugar _____   **Menstrual cycle phase** __pre __pms __have period

Today I physically feel:

_____

_____

*Today I mentally feel:*_____

_____

Any unusual activity or events: _____

_____

Food & Hydration:_____

_____

_____

Medical appointments, procedures or notes: _____

_____

DATE_____

Blood Pressure sitting ____/____   standing ____/____   Pulse _____BPM

Blood Sugar _____   **Menstrual cycle phase** __pre __pms __have period

Today I physically feel:

_____

_____

*Today I mentally feel:*_____

_____

Any unusual activity or events: _____

_____

Food & Hydration:_____

_____

_____

Medical appointments, procedures or notes: _____

_____

DATE_____

Blood Pressure sitting ____/____ standing ____/____ Pulse _____BPM

Blood Sugar _____ **Menstrual cycle phase** __pre __pms __have period

Today I physically feel:

_____

_____

*Today I mentally feel:*_____

_____

Any unusual activity or events: _____

_____

Food & Hydration:_____

_____

_____

Medical appointments, procedures or notes: _____

_____

DATE_____

Blood Pressure sitting ____/____ standing ____/____ Pulse _____BPM

Blood Sugar _____ **Menstrual cycle phase** __pre __pms __have period

Today I physically feel:

_____

_____

*Today I mentally feel:*_____

_____

Any unusual activity or events: _____

_____

Food & Hydration:_____

_____

_____

Medical appointments, procedures or notes: _____

_____

DATE_____

Blood Pressure sitting ____/____ standing ____/____ Pulse _____BPM

Blood Sugar _____ **Menstrual cycle phase** __pre __pms __have period

Today I physically feel:

_____

_____

*Today I mentally feel:*_____

_____

Any unusual activity or events: _____

_____

Food & Hydration:_____

_____

_____

Medical appointments, procedures or notes: _____

_____

DATE_____

Blood Pressure sitting ____/____   standing ____/____   Pulse _____BPM

Blood Sugar _____   **Menstrual cycle phase** __pre __pms __have period

Today I physically feel:

_____

_____

*Today I mentally feel:*_____

_____

Any unusual activity or events: _____

_____

Food & Hydration:_____

_____

_____

_____

Medical appointments, procedures or notes: _____

_____

DATE_____

Blood Pressure sitting ____/____ standing ____/____ Pulse _____BPM

Blood Sugar _____ **Menstrual cycle phase** __pre __pms __have period

Today I physically feel:

_____

_____

*Today I mentally feel:*_____

_____

Any unusual activity or events: _____

_____

Food & Hydration:_____

_____

_____

Medical appointments, procedures or notes: _____

_____

DATE_____

Blood Pressure sitting ____/____ standing ____/____ Pulse _____BPM

Blood Sugar _____ **Menstrual cycle phase** __pre __pms __have period

Today I physically feel:

_____

_____

*Today I mentally feel:*_____

_____

Any unusual activity or events: _____

_____

Food & Hydration:_____

_____

_____

Medical appointments, procedures or notes: _____

_____

DATE_____

Blood Pressure sitting ____/____ standing ____/____ Pulse _____BPM

Blood Sugar _____ **Menstrual cycle phase** __pre __pms __have period

Today I physically feel:

_____

_____

*Today I mentally feel:*_____

_____

Any unusual activity or events: _____

_____

Food & Hydration:_____

_____

_____

_____

Medical appointments, procedures or notes: _____

_____

DATE_____

Blood Pressure sitting ____/____ standing ____/____ Pulse _____BPM

Blood Sugar _____ **Menstrual cycle phase** __pre __pms __have period

Today I physically feel:

_____

_____

*Today I mentally feel:*_____

_____

Any unusual activity or events: _____

_____

Food & Hydration:_____

_____

_____

_____

Medical appointments, procedures or notes: _____

_____

DATE_____

Blood Pressure sitting ____/____   standing ____/____   Pulse _____BPM

Blood Sugar _____   **Menstrual cycle phase** __pre __pms __have period

Today I physically feel:

_____

_____

*Today I mentally feel:*_____

_____

Any unusual activity or events: _____

_____

Food & Hydration:_____

_____

_____

Medical appointments, procedures or notes: _____

_____

DATE_____

Blood Pressure   sitting ____/____   standing ____/____   Pulse _____BPM

Blood Sugar _____   **Menstrual cycle phase**   __pre   __pms   __have period

Today I physically feel:

_____

_____

*Today I mentally feel:*_____

_____

Any unusual activity or events: _____

_____

Food & Hydration:_____

_____

_____

Medical appointments, procedures or notes: _____

_____

What I have learned this month

_____

_____

_____

_____

_____

_____

_____

_____

_____

_____

_____

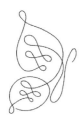

Month & Year

As of the first of the month, I am currently taking the following medications:

Name	Dosage	Frequency
_____	_____	_____
_____	_____	_____
_____	_____	_____
_____	_____	_____
_____	_____	_____
_____	_____	_____
_____	_____	_____

I have the following Dr. appointments and procedures scheduled:

_____

_____

_____

I have the following non-standard activities planned:

_____

_____

_____

DATE_____

Blood Pressure   sitting ____/____   standing ____/____   Pulse _____BPM

Blood Sugar _____   **Menstrual cycle phase** __pre __pms __have period

Today I physically feel:

_____

_____

*Today I mentally feel:*_____

_____

Any unusual activity or events: _____

_____

Food & Hydration:_____

_____

_____

_____

Medical appointments, procedures or notes: _____

_____

DATE_____

Blood Pressure sitting ____/____ standing ____/____ Pulse _____BPM

Blood Sugar _____ **Menstrual cycle phase** __pre __pms __have period

Today I physically feel:

_____

_____

*Today I mentally feel:*_____

_____

Any unusual activity or events: _____

_____

Food & Hydration:_____

_____

_____

_____

Medical appointments, procedures or notes: _____

_____

DATE_____

Blood Pressure   sitting ____/____   standing ____/____   Pulse _____BPM

Blood Sugar _____   **Menstrual cycle phase** __pre   __pms   __have period

Today I physically feel:

_____

_____

*Today I mentally feel:*_____

_____

Any unusual activity or events: _____

_____

Food & Hydration:_____

_____

_____

_____

Medical appointments, procedures or notes: _____

_____

DATE_____

Blood Pressure   sitting ____/____   standing ____/____   Pulse _____BPM

Blood Sugar _____   **Menstrual cycle phase** __pre __pms __have period

Today I physically feel:

_____

_____

*Today I mentally feel:*_____

_____

Any unusual activity or events: _____

_____

Food & Hydration:_____

_____

_____

Medical appointments, procedures or notes: _____

_____

DATE_____

Blood Pressure sitting ____/____   standing ____/____   Pulse _____BPM

Blood Sugar _____   **Menstrual cycle phase** __pre __pms __have period

Today I physically feel:

_____

_____

*Today I mentally feel:*_____

_____

Any unusual activity or events: _____

_____

Food & Hydration:_____

_____

_____

Medical appointments, procedures or notes: _____

_____

DATE_____

Blood Pressure sitting ____/____   standing ____/____   Pulse _____BPM

Blood Sugar _____   **Menstrual cycle phase** __pre __pms __have period

Today I physically feel:

_____

_____

*Today I mentally feel:*_____

_____

Any unusual activity or events: _____

_____

Food & Hydration:_____

_____

_____

_____

Medical appointments, procedures or notes: _____

_____

DATE_____

Blood Pressure sitting ____/____   standing ____/____   Pulse _____BPM

Blood Sugar _____   **Menstrual cycle phase** __pre __pms __have period

Today I physically feel:

_____

_____

*Today I mentally feel:*_____

_____

Any unusual activity or events: _____

_____

Food & Hydration:_____

_____

_____

Medical appointments, procedures or notes: _____

_____

DATE_____

Blood Pressure sitting ____/____ standing ____/____ Pulse _____BPM

Blood Sugar _____ **Menstrual cycle phase** __pre __pms __have period

Today I physically feel:

_____

_____

*Today I mentally feel:*_____

_____

Any unusual activity or events: _____

_____

Food & Hydration:_____

_____

_____

Medical appointments, procedures or notes: _____

_____

DATE_____

Blood Pressure   sitting ____/____   standing ____/____   Pulse _____BPM

Blood Sugar _____   **Menstrual cycle phase** __pre __pms __have period

Today I physically feel:

_____

_____

*Today I mentally feel:*_____

_____

Any unusual activity or events: _____

_____

Food & Hydration:_____

_____

_____

Medical appointments, procedures or notes: _____

_____

DATE_____

Blood Pressure sitting ____/____   standing ____/____   Pulse _____BPM

Blood Sugar _____   **Menstrual cycle phase** __pre __pms __have period

Today I physically feel:

_____

_____

*Today I mentally feel:*_____

_____

Any unusual activity or events: _____

_____

Food & Hydration:_____

_____

_____

_____

Medical appointments, procedures or notes: _____

_____

DATE_____

Blood Pressure sitting ____/____   standing ____/____   Pulse _____BPM

Blood Sugar _____   **Menstrual cycle phase** __pre __pms __have period

Today I physically feel:

_____

_____

*Today I mentally feel:*_____

_____

Any unusual activity or events: _____

_____

Food & Hydration:_____

_____

_____

_____

Medical appointments, procedures or notes: _____

_____

DATE_____

Blood Pressure sitting ____/____ standing ____/____ Pulse _____BPM

Blood Sugar _____ **Menstrual cycle phase** __pre __pms __have period

Today I physically feel:

_____

_____

*Today I mentally feel:*_____

_____

Any unusual activity or events: _____

_____

Food & Hydration:_____

_____

_____

Medical appointments, procedures or notes: _____

_____

DATE_____

Blood Pressure   sitting ____/____   standing ____/____   Pulse _____BPM

Blood Sugar _____   **Menstrual cycle phase** __pre   __pms   __have period

Today I physically feel:

_____

_____

*Today I mentally feel:*_____

_____

Any unusual activity or events: _____

_____

Food & Hydration:_____

_____

_____

_____

Medical appointments, procedures or notes: _____

_____

DATE_____

Blood Pressure   sitting ___/___   standing ___/___   Pulse ____BPM

Blood Sugar _____   **Menstrual cycle phase** __pre __pms __have period

Today I physically feel:

_____

_____

*Today I mentally feel:*_____

_____

Any unusual activity or events: _____

_____

Food & Hydration:_____

_____

_____

Medical appointments, procedures or notes: _____

_____

DATE_____

Blood Pressure sitting ____/____   standing ____/____   Pulse _____BPM

Blood Sugar _____   **Menstrual cycle phase** __pre __pms __have period

Today I physically feel:

_____

_____

*Today I mentally feel:*_____

_____

Any unusual activity or events: _____

_____

Food & Hydration:_____

_____

_____

_____

Medical appointments, procedures or notes: _____

_____

DATE_____

Blood Pressure   sitting ____/____   standing ____/____   Pulse _____BPM

Blood Sugar _____   **Menstrual cycle phase** __pre __pms __have period

Today I physically feel:

_____

_____

*Today I mentally feel:*_____

_____

Any unusual activity or events: _____

_____

Food & Hydration:_____

_____

_____

_____

Medical appointments, procedures or notes: _____

_____

DATE_____

Blood Pressure sitting ____/____   standing ____/____   Pulse _____BPM

Blood Sugar _____   **Menstrual cycle phase** __pre __pms __have period

Today I physically feel:

_____

_____

*Today I mentally feel:*_____

_____

Any unusual activity or events: _____

_____

Food & Hydration:_____

_____

_____

_____

Medical appointments, procedures or notes: _____

_____

DATE_____

Blood Pressure   sitting ____/____   standing ____/____   Pulse _____BPM

Blood Sugar _____   **Menstrual cycle phase** __pre __pms __have period

Today I physically feel:

_____

_____

*Today I mentally feel:*_____

_____

Any unusual activity or events: _____

_____

*Food & Hydration:*_____

_____

_____

Medical appointments, procedures or notes: _____

_____

DATE_____

Blood Pressure   sitting ____/____   standing ____/____   Pulse _____BPM

Blood Sugar _____   **Menstrual cycle phase** __pre   __pms   __have period

Today I physically feel:

_____

_____

*Today I mentally feel:*_____

_____

Any unusual activity or events: _____

_____

Food & Hydration:_____

_____

_____

_____

Medical appointments, procedures or notes: _____

_____

DATE_____

Blood Pressure   sitting ___/___   standing ___/___   Pulse _____BPM

Blood Sugar _____   **Menstrual cycle phase** __pre __pms __have period

Today I physically feel:

_____

_____

*Today I mentally feel:*_____

_____

Any unusual activity or events: _____

_____

*Food & Hydration:*_____

_____

_____

Medical appointments, procedures or notes: _____

_____

DATE_____

Blood Pressure sitting ____/____ standing ____/____ Pulse _____BPM

Blood Sugar _____ **Menstrual cycle phase** __pre __pms __have period

Today I physically feel:

_____

_____

*Today I mentally feel:*_____

_____

Any unusual activity or events: _____

_____

Food & Hydration:_____

_____

_____

Medical appointments, procedures or notes: _____

_____

DATE_____

Blood Pressure   sitting ____/____   standing ____/____   Pulse _____BPM

Blood Sugar _____   **Menstrual cycle phase**   __pre   __pms   __have period

Today I physically feel:

_____

_____

*Today I mentally feel:*_____

_____

Any unusual activity or events: _____

_____

Food & Hydration:_____

_____

_____

Medical appointments, procedures or notes: _____

_____

DATE_____

Blood Pressure   sitting ____/____   standing ____/____   Pulse _____BPM

Blood Sugar _____   **Menstrual cycle phase** __pre __pms __have period

Today I physically feel:

_____

_____

*Today I mentally feel:*_____

_____

Any unusual activity or events: _____

_____

Food & Hydration:_____

_____

_____

Medical appointments, procedures or notes: _____

_____

DATE_____

Blood Pressure sitting ____/____   standing ____/____   Pulse _____BPM

Blood Sugar _____   **Menstrual cycle phase** __pre __pms __have period

Today I physically feel:

_____

_____

*Today I mentally feel:*_____

_____

Any unusual activity or events: _____

_____

Food & Hydration:_____

_____

_____

_____

Medical appointments, procedures or notes: _____

_____

DATE_____

Blood Pressure   sitting ____/____   standing ____/____   Pulse _____BPM

Blood Sugar _____   **Menstrual cycle phase** __pre __pms __have period

Today I physically feel:

_____

_____

*Today I mentally feel:*_____

_____

Any unusual activity or events: _____

_____

Food & Hydration:_____

_____

_____

_____

Medical appointments, procedures or notes: _____

_____

DATE_____

Blood Pressure   sitting ____/____   standing ____/____   Pulse _____BPM

Blood Sugar _____   **Menstrual cycle phase** __pre __pms __have period

Today I physically feel:

_____

_____

*Today I mentally feel:*_____

_____

Any unusual activity or events: _____

_____

Food & Hydration:_____

_____

_____

_____

Medical appointments, procedures or notes: _____

_____

DATE_____

Blood Pressure sitting ____/____ standing ____/____ Pulse _____BPM

Blood Sugar _____ **Menstrual cycle phase** __pre __pms __have period

Today I physically feel:

_____

_____

*Today I mentally feel:*_____

_____

Any unusual activity or events: _____

_____

Food & Hydration:_____

_____

_____

Medical appointments, procedures or notes: _____

_____

DATE_____

Blood Pressure sitting ____/____ standing ____/____ Pulse _____BPM

Blood Sugar _____ **Menstrual cycle phase** __pre __pms __have period

Today I physically feel:

_____

_____

*Today I mentally feel:*_____

_____

Any unusual activity or events: _____

_____

Food & Hydration:_____

_____

_____

Medical appointments, procedures or notes: _____

_____

DATE_____

Blood Pressure sitting ____/____   standing ____/____   Pulse _____BPM

Blood Sugar _____   **Menstrual cycle phase** __pre __pms __have period

Today I physically feel:

_____

_____

*Today I mentally feel:*_____

_____

Any unusual activity or events: _____

_____

Food & Hydration:_____

_____

_____

Medical appointments, procedures or notes: _____

_____

DATE_____

Blood Pressure sitting ____/____ standing ____/____ Pulse _____BPM

Blood Sugar _____ **Menstrual cycle phase** __pre __pms __have period

Today I physically feel:

_____

_____

*Today I mentally feel:*_____

_____

Any unusual activity or events: _____

_____

Food & Hydration:_____

_____

_____

Medical appointments, procedures or notes: _____

_____

DATE_____

Blood Pressure   sitting ____/____   standing ____/____   Pulse _____BPM

Blood Sugar _____   **Menstrual cycle phase** __pre __pms __have period

Today I physically feel:

_____

_____

*Today I mentally feel:*_____

_____

Any unusual activity or events: _____

_____

Food & Hydration:_____

_____

_____

_____

Medical appointments, procedures or notes: _____

_____

What I have learned this month

_____

_____

_____

_____

_____

_____

_____

_____

_____

_____

_____

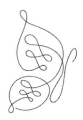

Month & Year

As of the first of the month, I am currently taking the following medications:

Name   Dosage   Frequency

_____   _____   _____

_____   _____   _____

_____   _____   _____

_____   _____   _____

_____   _____   _____

_____   _____   _____

_____   _____   _____

I have the following Dr. appointments and procedures scheduled:

_____

_____

_____

I have the following non-standard activities planned:

_____

_____

_____

DATE_____

Blood Pressure   sitting ____/____   standing ____/____   Pulse _____BPM

Blood Sugar _____   **Menstrual cycle phase** __pre __pms __have period

Today I physically feel:

_____

_____

*Today I mentally feel:*_____

_____

Any unusual activity or events: _____

_____

Food & Hydration:_____

_____

_____

_____

Medical appointments, procedures or notes: _____

_____

DATE_____

Blood Pressure   sitting ____/____   standing ____/____   Pulse _____BPM

Blood Sugar _____   **Menstrual cycle phase** __pre __pms __have period

Today I physically feel:

_____

_____

*Today I mentally feel:*_____

_____

Any unusual activity or events: _____

_____

Food & Hydration:_____

_____

_____

Medical appointments, procedures or notes: _____

_____

DATE_____

Blood Pressure   sitting ____/____   standing ____/____   Pulse _____BPM

Blood Sugar _____   **Menstrual cycle phase** __pre __pms __have period

Today I physically feel:

_____

_____

*Today I mentally feel:*_____

_____

Any unusual activity or events: _____

_____

Food & Hydration:_____

_____

_____

_____

Medical appointments, procedures or notes: _____

_____

DATE_____

Blood Pressure   sitting ____/____   standing ____/____   Pulse _____BPM

Blood Sugar _____   **Menstrual cycle phase**   __pre   __pms   __have period

Today I physically feel:

_____

_____

*Today I mentally feel:*_____

_____

Any unusual activity or events: _____

_____

Food & Hydration:_____

_____

_____

_____

Medical appointments, procedures or notes: _____

_____

DATE_____

Blood Pressure sitting ____/____   standing ____/____   Pulse _____BPM

Blood Sugar _____   **Menstrual cycle phase** __pre __pms __have period

Today I physically feel:

_____

_____

*Today I mentally feel:*_____

_____

Any unusual activity or events: _____

_____

Food & Hydration:_____

_____

_____

Medical appointments, procedures or notes: _____

_____

DATE_____

Blood Pressure sitting ____/____   standing ____/____   Pulse _____BPM

Blood Sugar _____   **Menstrual cycle phase** __pre __pms __have period

Today I physically feel:

_____

_____

*Today I mentally feel:*_____

_____

Any unusual activity or events: _____

_____

Food & Hydration:_____

_____

_____

Medical appointments, procedures or notes: _____

_____

DATE_____

Blood Pressure   sitting ____/____   standing ____/____   Pulse _____BPM

Blood Sugar _____   **Menstrual cycle phase** __pre __pms __have period

Today I physically feel:

_____

_____

*Today I mentally feel:*_____

_____

Any unusual activity or events: _____

_____

*Food & Hydration:*_____

_____

_____

_____

Medical appointments, procedures or notes: _____

_____

DATE_____

Blood Pressure sitting ____/____ standing ____/____ Pulse _____BPM

Blood Sugar _____ **Menstrual cycle phase** __pre __pms __have period

Today I physically feel:

_____

_____

*Today I mentally feel:*_____

_____

Any unusual activity or events: _____

_____

Food & Hydration:_____

_____

_____

_____

Medical appointments, procedures or notes: _____

_____

DATE_____

Blood Pressure sitting ____/____ standing ____/____ Pulse _____BPM

Blood Sugar _____ **Menstrual cycle phase** __pre __pms __have period

Today I physically feel:

_____

_____

*Today I mentally feel:*_____

_____

Any unusual activity or events: _____

_____

Food & Hydration:_____

_____

_____

_____

Medical appointments, procedures or notes: _____

_____

DATE_____

Blood Pressure sitting ____/____ standing ____/____ Pulse _____BPM

Blood Sugar _____ **Menstrual cycle phase** __pre __pms __have period

Today I physically feel:

_____

_____

*Today I mentally feel:*_____

_____

Any unusual activity or events: _____

_____

Food & Hydration:_____

_____

_____

Medical appointments, procedures or notes: _____

_____

DATE_____

Blood Pressure   sitting ____/____   standing ____/____   Pulse _____BPM

Blood Sugar _____   **Menstrual cycle phase** __pre __pms __have period

Today I physically feel:

_____

_____

*Today I mentally feel:*_____

_____

Any unusual activity or events: _____

_____

Food & Hydration:_____

_____

_____

_____

Medical appointments, procedures or notes: _____

_____

DATE_____

Blood Pressure sitting ____/____   standing ____/____   Pulse _____BPM

Blood Sugar _____   **Menstrual cycle phase** __pre __pms __have period

Today I physically feel:

_____

_____

*Today I mentally feel:*_____

_____

Any unusual activity or events: _____

_____

Food & Hydration:_____

_____

_____

_____

Medical appointments, procedures or notes: _____

_____

DATE_____

Blood Pressure sitting ____/____   standing ____/____   Pulse _____BPM

Blood Sugar _____   **Menstrual cycle phase** __pre __pms __have period

Today I physically feel:

_____

_____

*Today I mentally feel:*_____

_____

Any unusual activity or events: _____

_____

Food & Hydration:_____

_____

_____

_____

Medical appointments, procedures or notes: _____

_____

DATE_____

Blood Pressure   sitting ____/____   standing ____/____   Pulse _____BPM

Blood Sugar _____   **Menstrual cycle phase**   __pre   __pms   __have period

Today I physically feel:

_____

_____

*Today I mentally feel:*_____

_____

Any unusual activity or events: _____

_____

Food & Hydration:_____

_____

_____

_____

Medical appointments, procedures or notes: _____

_____

DATE_____

Blood Pressure   sitting ____/____   standing ____/____   Pulse _____BPM

Blood Sugar _____   **Menstrual cycle phase**   __pre   __pms   __have period

Today I physically feel:

_____

_____

*Today I mentally feel:*_____

_____

Any unusual activity or events: _____

_____

Food & Hydration:_____

_____

_____

_____

Medical appointments, procedures or notes: _____

_____

DATE_____

Blood Pressure   sitting ____/____   standing ____/____   Pulse _____BPM

Blood Sugar _____   **Menstrual cycle phase** __pre __pms __have period

Today I physically feel:

_____

_____

*Today I mentally feel:*_____

_____

Any unusual activity or events: _____

_____

Food & Hydration:_____

_____

_____

Medical appointments, procedures or notes: _____

_____

DATE_____

Blood Pressure sitting ____/____ standing ____/____ Pulse _____BPM

Blood Sugar _____ **Menstrual cycle phase** __pre __pms __have period

Today I physically feel:

_____

_____

*Today I mentally feel:*_____

_____

Any unusual activity or events: _____

_____

Food & Hydration:_____

_____

_____

_____

Medical appointments, procedures or notes: _____

_____

DATE_____

Blood Pressure   sitting ____/____   standing ____/____   Pulse _____BPM

Blood Sugar _____   **Menstrual cycle phase** __pre   __pms   __have period

Today I physically feel:

_____

_____

*Today I mentally feel:*_____

_____

Any unusual activity or events: _____

_____

Food & Hydration:_____

_____

_____

_____

Medical appointments, procedures or notes: _____

_____

DATE_____

Blood Pressure   sitting ____/____   standing ____/____   Pulse _____BPM

Blood Sugar _____   **Menstrual cycle phase** __pre __pms __have period

Today I physically feel:

_____

_____

*Today I mentally feel:*_____

_____

Any unusual activity or events: _____

_____

Food & Hydration:_____

_____

_____

_____

Medical appointments, procedures or notes: _____

_____

DATE_____

Blood Pressure sitting ____/____ standing ____/____ Pulse _____BPM

Blood Sugar _____ **Menstrual cycle phase** __pre __pms __have period

Today I physically feel:

_____

_____

*Today I mentally feel:*_____

_____

Any unusual activity or events: _____

_____

Food & Hydration:_____

_____

_____

Medical appointments, procedures or notes: _____

_____

DATE_____

Blood Pressure sitting ____/____   standing ____/____   Pulse _____BPM

Blood Sugar _____   **Menstrual cycle phase** __pre __pms __have period

Today I physically feel:

_____

_____

*Today I mentally feel:*_____

_____

Any unusual activity or events: _____

_____

Food & Hydration:_____

_____

_____

Medical appointments, procedures or notes: _____

_____

DATE_____

Blood Pressure sitting ____/____ standing ____/____ Pulse _____BPM

Blood Sugar _____ **Menstrual cycle phase** __pre __pms __have period

Today I physically feel:

_____

_____

*Today I mentally feel:*_____

_____

Any unusual activity or events: _____

_____

Food & Hydration:_____

_____

_____

Medical appointments, procedures or notes: _____

_____

DATE_____

Blood Pressure sitting _____/_____ standing _____/_____ Pulse _____BPM

Blood Sugar _____   **Menstrual cycle phase** __pre __pms __have period

Today I physically feel:

_____

_____

*Today I mentally feel:*_____

_____

Any unusual activity or events: _____

_____

Food & Hydration:_____

_____

_____

Medical appointments, procedures or notes: _____

_____

DATE_____

Blood Pressure sitting ____/____   standing ____/____   Pulse _____BPM

Blood Sugar _____   **Menstrual cycle phase** __pre   __pms   __have period

Today I physically feel:

_____

_____

*Today I mentally feel:*_____

_____

Any unusual activity or events: _____

_____

Food & Hydration:_____

_____

_____

Medical appointments, procedures or notes: _____

_____

DATE_____

Blood Pressure sitting ____/____ standing ____/____ Pulse _____BPM

Blood Sugar _____ **Menstrual cycle phase** __pre __pms __have period

Today I physically feel:

_____

_____

*Today I mentally feel:*_____

_____

Any unusual activity or events: _____

_____

*Food & Hydration:*_____

_____

_____

_____

Medical appointments, procedures or notes: _____

_____

DATE_____

Blood Pressure   sitting ____/____   standing ____/____   Pulse _____BPM

Blood Sugar _____   **Menstrual cycle phase** __pre __pms __have period

Today I physically feel:

_____

_____

*Today I mentally feel:*_____

_____

Any unusual activity or events: _____

_____

Food & Hydration:_____

_____

_____

_____

Medical appointments, procedures or notes: _____

_____

DATE_____

Blood Pressure   sitting ____/____   standing ____/____   Pulse _____BPM

Blood Sugar _____   **Menstrual cycle phase**   __pre   __pms   __have period

Today I physically feel:

_____

_____

*Today I mentally feel:*_____

_____

Any unusual activity or events: _____

_____

Food & Hydration:_____

_____

_____

Medical appointments, procedures or notes: _____

_____

DATE_____

Blood Pressure   sitting ____/____   standing ____/____   Pulse _____BPM

Blood Sugar _____   **Menstrual cycle phase** __pre   __pms   __have period

Today I physically feel:

_____

_____

*Today I mentally feel:*_____

_____

Any unusual activity or events: _____

_____

Food & Hydration:_____

_____

_____

_____

Medical appointments, procedures or notes: _____

_____

DATE_____

Blood Pressure   sitting ___/___   standing ___/___   Pulse _____BPM

Blood Sugar _____   **Menstrual cycle phase**   __pre   __pms   __have period

Today I physically feel:

_____

_____

*Today I mentally feel:*_____

_____

Any unusual activity or events: _____

_____

Food & Hydration:_____

_____

_____

Medical appointments, procedures or notes: _____

_____

DATE_____

Blood Pressure sitting ____/____ standing ____/____ Pulse _____BPM

Blood Sugar _____ **Menstrual cycle phase** __pre __pms __have period

Today I physically feel:

_____

_____

*Today I mentally feel:*_____

_____

Any unusual activity or events: _____

_____

Food & Hydration:_____

_____

_____

_____

Medical appointments, procedures or notes: _____

_____

DATE_____

Blood Pressure sitting ____/____   standing ____/____   Pulse _____BPM

Blood Sugar _____   **Menstrual cycle phase** __pre   __pms   __have period

Today I physically feel:

_____

_____

*Today I mentally feel:*_____

_____

Any unusual activity or events: _____

_____

Food & Hydration:_____

_____

_____

_____

Medical appointments, procedures or notes: _____

_____

What I have learned this month

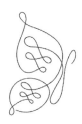

Month & Year

As of the first of the month, I am currently taking the following medications:

Name	Dosage	Frequency
_____	_____	_____
_____	_____	_____
_____	_____	_____
_____	_____	_____
_____	_____	_____
_____	_____	_____
_____	_____	_____

I have the following Dr. appointments and procedures scheduled:

_____

_____

_____

I have the following non-standard activities planned:

_____

_____

_____

DATE_____

Blood Pressure   sitting ____/____   standing ____/____   Pulse _____BPM

Blood Sugar _____   **Menstrual cycle phase**   __pre   __pms   __have period

Today I physically feel:

_____

_____

*Today I mentally feel:*_____

_____

Any unusual activity or events: _____

_____

Food & Hydration:_____

_____

_____

_____

Medical appointments, procedures or notes: _____

_____

DATE_____

Blood Pressure sitting ____/____ standing ____/____ Pulse _____BPM

Blood Sugar _____ **Menstrual cycle phase** ___pre ___pms ___have period

Today I physically feel:

_____

_____

*Today I mentally feel:*_____

_____

Any unusual activity or events: _____

_____

Food & Hydration:_____

_____

_____

_____

Medical appointments, procedures or notes: _____

_____

DATE_____

Blood Pressure sitting ____/____   standing ____/____   Pulse _____BPM

Blood Sugar _____   **Menstrual cycle phase** __pre __pms __have period

Today I physically feel:

_____

_____

*Today I mentally feel:*_____

_____

Any unusual activity or events: _____

_____

Food & Hydration:_____

_____

_____

_____

Medical appointments, procedures or notes: _____

_____

DATE_____

Blood Pressure sitting ____/____   standing ____/____   Pulse _____BPM

Blood Sugar _____   **Menstrual cycle phase** __pre __pms __have period

Today I physically feel:

_____

_____

*Today I mentally feel:*_____

_____

Any unusual activity or events: _____

_____

Food & Hydration:_____

_____

_____

Medical appointments, procedures or notes: _____

_____

DATE_____

Blood Pressure sitting ____/____   standing ____/____   Pulse _____BPM

Blood Sugar _____   **Menstrual cycle phase** __pre __pms __have period

Today I physically feel:

_____

_____

*Today I mentally feel:*_____

_____

Any unusual activity or events: _____

_____

Food & Hydration:_____

_____

_____

Medical appointments, procedures or notes: _____

_____

DATE_____

Blood Pressure   sitting ____/____   standing ____/____   Pulse _____BPM

Blood Sugar _____   **Menstrual cycle phase** __pre __pms __have period

Today I physically feel:

_____

_____

*Today I mentally feel:*_____

_____

Any unusual activity or events: _____

_____

Food & Hydration:_____

_____

_____

Medical appointments, procedures or notes: _____

_____

DATE_____

Blood Pressure sitting ____/____ standing ____/____ Pulse _____BPM

Blood Sugar _____ **Menstrual cycle phase** __pre __pms __have period

Today I physically feel:

_____

_____

*Today I mentally feel:*_____

_____

Any unusual activity or events: _____

_____

Food & Hydration:_____

_____

_____

_____

Medical appointments, procedures or notes: _____

_____

DATE_____

Blood Pressure sitting ____/____   standing ____/____   Pulse _____BPM

Blood Sugar _____   **Menstrual cycle phase** __pre __pms __have period

Today I physically feel:

_____

_____

*Today I mentally feel:*_____

_____

Any unusual activity or events: _____

_____

Food & Hydration:_____

_____

_____

Medical appointments, procedures or notes: _____

_____

DATE_____

Blood Pressure   sitting ____/____   standing ____/____   Pulse _____BPM

Blood Sugar _____   **Menstrual cycle phase** __pre   __pms   __have period

Today I physically feel:

_____

_____

*Today I mentally feel:*_____

_____

Any unusual activity or events: _____

_____

Food & Hydration:_____

_____

_____

Medical appointments, procedures or notes: _____

_____

DATE_____

Blood Pressure sitting ____/____ standing ____/____ Pulse _____BPM

Blood Sugar _____ **Menstrual cycle phase** __pre __pms __have period

Today I physically feel:

_____

_____

*Today I mentally feel:*_____

_____

Any unusual activity or events: _____

_____

Food & Hydration:_____

_____

_____

Medical appointments, procedures or notes: _____

_____

DATE_____

Blood Pressure   sitting ___/___   standing ___/___   Pulse ____BPM

Blood Sugar ____   **Menstrual cycle phase** __pre __pms __have period

Today I physically feel:

_____

_____

*Today I mentally feel:*_____

_____

Any unusual activity or events: _____

_____

Food & Hydration:_____

_____

_____

Medical appointments, procedures or notes: _____

_____

DATE_____

Blood Pressure sitting ____/____ standing ____/____ Pulse _____BPM

Blood Sugar _____ **Menstrual cycle phase** __pre __pms __have period

Today I physically feel:

_____

_____

*Today I mentally feel:*_____

_____

Any unusual activity or events: _____

_____

Food & Hydration:_____

_____

_____

_____

Medical appointments, procedures or notes: _____

_____

DATE_____

Blood Pressure sitting ____/____   standing ____/____   Pulse _____BPM

Blood Sugar _____   **Menstrual cycle phase** __pre __pms __have period

Today I physically feel:

_____

_____

*Today I mentally feel:*_____

_____

Any unusual activity or events: _____

_____

Food & Hydration:_____

_____

_____

Medical appointments, procedures or notes: _____

_____

DATE_____

Blood Pressure   sitting ____/____   standing ____/____   Pulse _____BPM

Blood Sugar _____   **Menstrual cycle phase**   __pre   __pms   __have period

Today I physically feel:

_____

_____

*Today I mentally feel:*_____

_____

Any unusual activity or events: _____

_____

Food & Hydration:_____

_____

_____

_____

Medical appointments, procedures or notes: _____

_____

DATE_____

Blood Pressure sitting ____/____   standing ____/____   Pulse _____BPM

Blood Sugar _____   **Menstrual cycle phase** __pre   __pms   __have period

Today I physically feel:

_____

_____

*Today I mentally feel:*_____

_____

Any unusual activity or events: _____

_____

*Food & Hydration:*_____

_____

_____

_____

Medical appointments, procedures or notes: _____

_____

DATE_____

Blood Pressure   sitting ____/____   standing ____/____   Pulse _____BPM

Blood Sugar _____   **Menstrual cycle phase** __pre __pms __have period

Today I physically feel:

_____

_____

*Today I mentally feel:*_____

_____

Any unusual activity or events: _____

_____

Food & Hydration:_____

_____

_____

Medical appointments, procedures or notes: _____

_____

DATE_____

Blood Pressure sitting ____/____   standing ____/____   Pulse _____BPM

Blood Sugar _____   **Menstrual cycle phase** __pre __pms __have period

Today I physically feel:

_____

_____

*Today I mentally feel:*_____

_____

Any unusual activity or events: _____

_____

Food & Hydration:_____

_____

_____

_____

Medical appointments, procedures or notes: _____

_____

DATE_____

Blood Pressure sitting ____/____ standing ____/____ Pulse _____BPM

Blood Sugar _____ **Menstrual cycle phase** __pre __pms __have period

Today I physically feel:

_____

_____

*Today I mentally feel:*_____

_____

Any unusual activity or events: _____

_____

Food & Hydration:_____

_____

_____

_____

Medical appointments, procedures or notes: _____

_____

DATE_____

Blood Pressure sitting ____/____ standing ____/____ Pulse _____BPM

Blood Sugar _____ **Menstrual cycle phase** __pre __pms __have period

Today I physically feel:

_____

_____

*Today I mentally feel:*_____

_____

Any unusual activity or events: _____

_____

Food & Hydration:_____

_____

_____

Medical appointments, procedures or notes: _____

_____

DATE_____

Blood Pressure sitting ____/____ standing ____/____ Pulse _____BPM

Blood Sugar _____ **Menstrual cycle phase** __pre __pms __have period

Today I physically feel:

_____

_____

*Today I mentally feel:*_____

_____

Any unusual activity or events: _____

_____

*Food & Hydration:*_____

_____

_____

_____

Medical appointments, procedures or notes: _____

_____

DATE_____

Blood Pressure sitting ____/____   standing ____/____   Pulse _____BPM

Blood Sugar _____   **Menstrual cycle phase** __pre __pms __have period

Today I physically feel:

_____

_____

*Today I mentally feel:*_____

_____

Any unusual activity or events: _____

_____

Food & Hydration:_____

_____

_____

_____

Medical appointments, procedures or notes: _____

_____

DATE_____

Blood Pressure   sitting ____/____   standing ____/____   Pulse _____BPM

Blood Sugar _____   **Menstrual cycle phase** __pre   __pms   __have period

Today I physically feel:

_____

_____

*Today I mentally feel:*_____

_____

Any unusual activity or events: _____

_____

Food & Hydration:_____

_____

_____

Medical appointments, procedures or notes: _____

_____

DATE_____

Blood Pressure sitting ____/____ standing ____/____ Pulse _____BPM

Blood Sugar _____ **Menstrual cycle phase** __pre __pms __have period

Today I physically feel:

_____

_____

*Today I mentally feel:*_____

_____

Any unusual activity or events: _____

_____

Food & Hydration:_____

_____

_____

_____

Medical appointments, procedures or notes: _____

_____

DATE_____

Blood Pressure sitting ____/____   standing ____/____   Pulse _____BPM

Blood Sugar _____   **Menstrual cycle phase** __pre __pms __have period

Today I physically feel:

_____

_____

*Today I mentally feel:*_____

_____

Any unusual activity or events: _____

_____

Food & Hydration:_____

_____

_____

Medical appointments, procedures or notes: _____

_____

DATE_____

Blood Pressure sitting ____/____ standing ____/____ Pulse _____BPM

Blood Sugar _____ **Menstrual cycle phase** __pre __pms __have period

Today I physically feel:

_____

_____

*Today I mentally feel:*_____

_____

Any unusual activity or events: _____

_____

Food & Hydration:_____

_____

_____

_____

Medical appointments, procedures or notes: _____

_____

DATE_____

Blood Pressure   sitting ____/____   standing ____/____   Pulse _____BPM

Blood Sugar _____   **Menstrual cycle phase** __pre __pms __have period

Today I physically feel:

_____

_____

*Today I mentally feel:*_____

_____

Any unusual activity or events: _____

_____

Food & Hydration:_____

_____

_____

Medical appointments, procedures or notes: _____

_____

DATE_____

Blood Pressure   sitting ____/____   standing ____/____   Pulse _____BPM

Blood Sugar _____   **Menstrual cycle phase** __pre   __pms   __have period

Today I physically feel:

_____

_____

*Today I mentally feel:*_____

_____

Any unusual activity or events: _____

_____

Food & Hydration:_____

_____

_____

_____

Medical appointments, procedures or notes: _____

_____

DATE_____

Blood Pressure sitting ___/___ standing ___/___ Pulse _____BPM

Blood Sugar _____   **Menstrual cycle phase** __pre __pms __have period

Today I physically feel:

_____

_____

*Today I mentally feel:*_____

_____

Any unusual activity or events: _____

_____

Food & Hydration:_____

_____

_____

_____

Medical appointments, procedures or notes: _____

_____

DATE_____

Blood Pressure sitting ____/____   standing ____/____   Pulse _____BPM

Blood Sugar _____   **Menstrual cycle phase** __pre __pms __have period

Today I physically feel:

_____

_____

*Today I mentally feel:*_____

_____

Any unusual activity or events: _____

_____

Food & Hydration:_____

_____

_____

_____

Medical appointments, procedures or notes: _____

_____

DATE_____

Blood Pressure   sitting ____/____   standing ____/____   Pulse _____BPM

Blood Sugar _____   **Menstrual cycle phase**   __pre   __pms   __have period

Today I physically feel:

_____

_____

*Today I mentally feel:*_____

_____

Any unusual activity or events: _____

_____

Food & Hydration:_____

_____

_____

Medical appointments, procedures or notes: _____

_____

DATE_____

Blood Pressure sitting ____/____   standing ____/____   Pulse _____BPM

Blood Sugar _____   **Menstrual cycle phase** __pre __pms __have period

Today I physically feel:

_____

_____

*Today I mentally feel:*_____

_____

Any unusual activity or events: _____

_____

Food & Hydration:_____

_____

_____

_____

Medical appointments, procedures or notes: _____

_____

What I have learned this month

_____

_____

_____

_____

_____

_____

_____

_____

_____

_____

_____

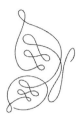

Month & Year

As of the first of the month, I am currently taking the following medications:

Name   Dosage   Frequency

_____   _____   _____

_____   _____   _____

_____   _____   _____

_____   _____   _____

_____   _____   _____

_____   _____   _____

I have the following Dr. appointments and procedures scheduled:

_____

_____

_____

I have the following non-standard activities planned:

_____

_____

_____

DATE_____

Blood Pressure sitting ____/____ standing ____/____ Pulse _____BPM

Blood Sugar _____   **Menstrual cycle phase** __pre __pms __have period

Today I physically feel:

_____

_____

*Today I mentally feel:*_____

_____

Any unusual activity or events: _____

_____

Food & Hydration:_____

_____

_____

_____

Medical appointments, procedures or notes: _____

_____

DATE_____

Blood Pressure   sitting ____/____   standing ____/____   Pulse _____BPM

Blood Sugar _____   **Menstrual cycle phase**   __pre   __pms   __have period

Today I physically feel:

_____

_____

*Today I mentally feel:*_____

_____

Any unusual activity or events: _____

_____

Food & Hydration:_____

_____

_____

_____

Medical appointments, procedures or notes: _____

_____

DATE_____

Blood Pressure sitting _____/_____   standing _____/_____   Pulse _____BPM

Blood Sugar _____   **Menstrual cycle phase** ___pre ___pms ___have period

Today I physically feel:

_____

_____

*Today I mentally feel:*_____

_____

Any unusual activity or events: _____

_____

Food & Hydration:_____

_____

_____

_____

Medical appointments, procedures or notes: _____

_____

DATE_____

Blood Pressure   sitting ____/____   standing ____/____   Pulse _____BPM

Blood Sugar _____   **Menstrual cycle phase** __pre __pms __have period

Today I physically feel:

_____

_____

*Today I mentally feel:*_____

_____

Any unusual activity or events: _____

_____

Food & Hydration:_____

_____

_____

_____

Medical appointments, procedures or notes: _____

_____

DATE_____

Blood Pressure sitting ____/____   standing ____/____   Pulse _____BPM

Blood Sugar _____   **Menstrual cycle phase** __pre __pms __have period

Today I physically feel:

_____

_____

*Today I mentally feel:*_____

_____

Any unusual activity or events: _____

_____

Food & Hydration:_____

_____

_____

Medical appointments, procedures or notes: _____

_____

DATE_____

Blood Pressure   sitting ____/____   standing ____/____   Pulse _____BPM

Blood Sugar _____   **Menstrual cycle phase** __pre __pms __have period

Today I physically feel:

_____

_____

*Today I mentally feel:*_____

_____

Any unusual activity or events: _____

_____

Food & Hydration:_____

_____

_____

_____

Medical appointments, procedures or notes: _____

_____

DATE_____

Blood Pressure   sitting ____/____   standing ____/____   Pulse _____BPM

Blood Sugar _____   **Menstrual cycle phase**   __pre   __pms   __have period

Today I physically feel:

_____

_____

*Today I mentally feel:*_____

_____

Any unusual activity or events: _____

_____

Food & Hydration:_____

_____

_____

_____

Medical appointments, procedures or notes: _____

_____

DATE_____

Blood Pressure sitting ____/____ standing ____/____ Pulse _____BPM

Blood Sugar _____ **Menstrual cycle phase** __pre __pms __have period

Today I physically feel:

_____

_____

*Today I mentally feel:*_____

_____

Any unusual activity or events: _____

_____

Food & Hydration:_____

_____

_____

_____

Medical appointments, procedures or notes: _____

_____

DATE_____

Blood Pressure sitting ____/____ standing ____/____ Pulse _____BPM

Blood Sugar _____ **Menstrual cycle phase** __pre __pms __have period

Today I physically feel:

_____

_____

*Today I mentally feel:*_____

_____

Any unusual activity or events: _____

_____

Food & Hydration:_____

_____

_____

_____

Medical appointments, procedures or notes: _____

_____

DATE_____

Blood Pressure   sitting ____/____   standing ____/____   Pulse _____BPM

Blood Sugar _____   **Menstrual cycle phase** __pre   __pms   __have period

Today I physically feel:

_____

_____

*Today I mentally feel:*_____

_____

Any unusual activity or events: _____

_____

Food & Hydration:_____

_____

_____

_____

Medical appointments, procedures or notes: _____

_____

DATE_____

Blood Pressure sitting ____/____ standing ____/____ Pulse _____BPM

Blood Sugar _____ **Menstrual cycle phase** __pre __pms __have period

Today I physically feel:

_____

_____

*Today I mentally feel:*_____

_____

Any unusual activity or events: _____

_____

Food & Hydration:_____

_____

_____

_____

Medical appointments, procedures or notes: _____

_____

DATE_____

Blood Pressure sitting ____/____   standing ____/____   Pulse _____BPM

Blood Sugar _____   **Menstrual cycle phase** __pre __pms __have period

Today I physically feel:

_____

_____

*Today I mentally feel:*_____

_____

Any unusual activity or events: _____

_____

Food & Hydration:_____

_____

_____

_____

Medical appointments, procedures or notes: _____

_____

DATE_____

Blood Pressure sitting ____/____ standing ____/____ Pulse _____BPM

Blood Sugar _____ **Menstrual cycle phase** __pre __pms __have period

Today I physically feel:

_____

_____

*Today I mentally feel:*_____

_____

Any unusual activity or events: _____

_____

Food & Hydration:_____

_____

_____

Medical appointments, procedures or notes: _____

_____

DATE_____

Blood Pressure   sitting ____/____   standing ____/____   Pulse _____BPM

Blood Sugar _____   **Menstrual cycle phase** __pre   __pms   __have period

Today I physically feel:

_____

_____

*Today I mentally feel:*_____

_____

Any unusual activity or events: _____

_____

Food & Hydration:_____

_____

_____

_____

Medical appointments, procedures or notes: _____

_____

DATE_____

Blood Pressure sitting ____/____   standing ____/____   Pulse _____BPM

Blood Sugar _____   **Menstrual cycle phase** __pre __pms __have period

Today I physically feel:

_____

_____

*Today I mentally feel:*_____

_____

Any unusual activity or events: _____

_____

Food & Hydration:_____

_____

_____

Medical appointments, procedures or notes: _____

_____

DATE_____

Blood Pressure sitting ____/____   standing ____/____   Pulse _____BPM

Blood Sugar _____   **Menstrual cycle phase** __pre __pms __have period

Today I physically feel:

_____

_____

*Today I mentally feel:*_____

_____

Any unusual activity or events: _____

_____

Food & Hydration:_____

_____

_____

_____

Medical appointments, procedures or notes: _____

_____

DATE_____

Blood Pressure   sitting ____/____   standing ____/____   Pulse _____BPM

Blood Sugar _____   **Menstrual cycle phase**   __pre   __pms   __have period

Today I physically feel:

_____

_____

*Today I mentally feel:*_____

_____

Any unusual activity or events: _____

_____

Food & Hydration:_____

_____

_____

Medical appointments, procedures or notes: _____

_____

DATE_____

Blood Pressure sitting ____/____ standing ____/____ Pulse _____BPM

Blood Sugar _____ **Menstrual cycle phase** __pre __pms __have period

Today I physically feel:

_____

_____

*Today I mentally feel:*_____

_____

Any unusual activity or events: _____

_____

Food & Hydration:_____

_____

_____

_____

Medical appointments, procedures or notes: _____

_____

DATE_____

Blood Pressure sitting ____/____ standing ____/____ Pulse _____BPM

Blood Sugar _____ **Menstrual cycle phase** __pre __pms __have period

Today I physically feel:

_____

_____

*Today I mentally feel:*_____

_____

Any unusual activity or events: _____

_____

Food & Hydration:_____

_____

_____

_____

Medical appointments, procedures or notes: _____

_____

DATE_____

Blood Pressure   sitting ____/____   standing ____/____   Pulse _____BPM

Blood Sugar _____   **Menstrual cycle phase** __pre __pms __have period

Today I physically feel:

_____

_____

*Today I mentally feel:*_____

_____

Any unusual activity or events: _____

_____

Food & Hydration:_____

_____

_____

_____

Medical appointments, procedures or notes: _____

_____

DATE_____

Blood Pressure sitting ____/____ standing ____/____ Pulse _____BPM

Blood Sugar _____ **Menstrual cycle phase** __pre __pms __have period

Today I physically feel:

_____,_____

_____

*Today I mentally feel:*_____

_____

Any unusual activity or events: _____

_____

Food & Hydration:_____

_____

_____

Medical appointments, procedures or notes: _____

_____

DATE_____

Blood Pressure   sitting ____/____   standing ____/____   Pulse _____BPM

Blood Sugar _____   **Menstrual cycle phase** __pre __pms __have period

Today I physically feel:

_____

_____

*Today I mentally feel:*_____

_____

Any unusual activity or events: _____

_____

Food & Hydration:_____

_____

_____

_____

Medical appointments, procedures or notes: _____

_____

DATE_____

Blood Pressure   sitting ____/____   standing ____/____   Pulse _____BPM

Blood Sugar _____   **Menstrual cycle phase** __pre __pms __have period

Today I physically feel:

_____

_____

*Today I mentally feel:*_____

_____

Any unusual activity or events: _____

_____

Food & Hydration:_____

_____

_____

Medical appointments, procedures or notes: _____

_____

DATE_____

Blood Pressure   sitting ____/____   standing ____/____   Pulse _____BPM

Blood Sugar _____   **Menstrual cycle phase** __pre __pms __have period

Today I physically feel:

_____

_____

*Today I mentally feel:*_____

_____

Any unusual activity or events: _____

_____

Food & Hydration:_____

_____

_____

_____

Medical appointments, procedures or notes: _____

_____

DATE_____

Blood Pressure sitting ____/____   standing ____/____   Pulse _____BPM

Blood Sugar _____   **Menstrual cycle phase** __pre __pms __have period

Today I physically feel:

_____

_____

*Today I mentally feel:*_____

_____

Any unusual activity or events: _____

_____

Food & Hydration:_____

_____

_____

_____

Medical appointments, procedures or notes: _____

_____

DATE_____

Blood Pressure sitting ____/____ standing ____/____ Pulse _____BPM

Blood Sugar _____ **Menstrual cycle phase** __pre __pms __have period

Today I physically feel:

_____

_____

*Today I mentally feel:*_____

_____

Any unusual activity or events: _____

_____

Food & Hydration:_____

_____

_____

Medical appointments, procedures or notes: _____

_____

DATE_____

Blood Pressure   sitting ____/____   standing ____/____   Pulse _____BPM

Blood Sugar _____   **Menstrual cycle phase** __pre __pms __have period

Today I physically feel:

_____

_____

*Today I mentally feel:*_____

_____

Any unusual activity or events: _____

_____

Food & Hydration:_____

_____

_____

_____

Medical appointments, procedures or notes: _____

_____

DATE_____

Blood Pressure   sitting ____/____   standing ____/____   Pulse _____BPM

Blood Sugar _____   **Menstrual cycle phase** __pre   __pms   __have period

Today I physically feel:

_____

_____

*Today I mentally feel:*_____

_____

Any unusual activity or events: _____

_____

Food & Hydration:_____

_____

_____

_____

Medical appointments, procedures or notes: _____

_____

DATE_____

Blood Pressure   sitting ____/____   standing ____/____   Pulse _____BPM

Blood Sugar _____   **Menstrual cycle phase** __pre __pms __have period

Today I physically feel:

_____

_____

*Today I mentally feel:*_____

_____

Any unusual activity or events: _____

_____

Food & Hydration:_____

_____

_____

_____

Medical appointments, procedures or notes: _____

_____

DATE_____

Blood Pressure   sitting ____/____   standing ____/____   Pulse _____BPM

Blood Sugar _____   **Menstrual cycle phase** __pre __pms __have period

Today I physically feel:

_____

_____

*Today I mentally feel:*_____

_____

Any unusual activity or events: _____

_____

Food & Hydration:_____

_____

_____

_____

Medical appointments, procedures or notes: _____

_____

DATE_____

Blood Pressure sitting ____/____ standing ____/____ Pulse _____BPM

Blood Sugar _____ **Menstrual cycle phase** __pre __pms __have period

Today I physically feel:

_____

_____

*Today I mentally feel:*_____

_____

Any unusual activity or events: _____

_____

Food & Hydration:_____

_____

_____

Medical appointments, procedures or notes: _____

_____

What I have learned this month

_____

_____

_____

_____

_____

_____

_____

_____

_____

_____

_____

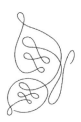

Month & Year

⟋⟋⟋⟋⟋⟋⟋⟋⟋⟋⟋⟋⟋⟋⟋⟋⟋⟋⟋⟋

As of the first of the month, I am currently taking the following medications:

Name	Dosage	Frequency
_____	_____	_____
_____	_____	_____
_____	_____	_____
_____	_____	_____
_____	_____	_____
_____	_____	_____
_____	_____	_____

I have the following Dr. appointments and procedures scheduled:

_____

_____

_____

I have the following non-standard activities planned:

_____

_____

_____

DATE_____

Blood Pressure   sitting ____/____   standing ____/____   Pulse _____BPM

Blood Sugar _____   **Menstrual cycle phase** __pre __pms __have period

Today I physically feel:

_____

_____

*Today I mentally feel:*_____

_____

Any unusual activity or events: _____

_____

Food & Hydration:_____

_____

_____

_____

Medical appointments, procedures or notes: _____

_____

DATE_____

Blood Pressure   sitting _____/_____   standing _____/_____   Pulse _____BPM

Blood Sugar _____   **Menstrual cycle phase**   __pre   __pms   __have period

Today I physically feel:

_____

_____

*Today I mentally feel:*_____

_____

Any unusual activity or events: _____

_____

Food & Hydration:_____

_____

_____

_____

Medical appointments, procedures or notes: _____

_____

DATE_____

Blood Pressure   sitting ____/____   standing ____/____   Pulse _____BPM

Blood Sugar _____   **Menstrual cycle phase** __pre   __pms   __have period

Today I physically feel:

_____

_____

*Today I mentally feel:*_____

_____

Any unusual activity or events: _____

_____

Food & Hydration:_____

_____

_____

_____

Medical appointments, procedures or notes: _____

_____

DATE_____

Blood Pressure sitting ____/____   standing ____/____   Pulse _____BPM

Blood Sugar _____   **Menstrual cycle phase** __pre __pms __have period

Today I physically feel:

_____

_____

*Today I mentally feel:*_____

_____

Any unusual activity or events: _____

_____

Food & Hydration:_____

_____

_____

_____

Medical appointments, procedures or notes: _____

_____

DATE_____

Blood Pressure sitting ____/____ standing ____/____ Pulse _____BPM

Blood Sugar _____ **Menstrual cycle phase** __pre __pms __have period

Today I physically feel:

_____

_____

*Today I mentally feel:*_____

_____

Any unusual activity or events: _____

_____

Food & Hydration:_____

_____

_____

_____

Medical appointments, procedures or notes: _____

_____

DATE_____

Blood Pressure sitting _____/_____   standing _____/_____   Pulse _____BPM

Blood Sugar _____   **Menstrual cycle phase** __pre __pms __have period

Today I physically feel:

_____

_____

*Today I mentally feel:*_____

_____

Any unusual activity or events: _____

_____

Food & Hydration:_____

_____

_____

_____

Medical appointments, procedures or notes: _____

_____

DATE_____

Blood Pressure sitting ____/____   standing ____/____   Pulse _____BPM

Blood Sugar _____   **Menstrual cycle phase** __pre __pms __have period

Today I physically feel:

_____

_____

*Today I mentally feel:*_____

_____

Any unusual activity or events: _____

_____

Food & Hydration:_____

_____

_____

Medical appointments, procedures or notes: _____

_____

DATE_____

Blood Pressure sitting ____/____   standing ____/____   Pulse _____BPM

Blood Sugar _____   **Menstrual cycle phase** __pre __pms __have period

Today I physically feel:

_____

_____

*Today I mentally feel:*_____

_____

Any unusual activity or events: _____

_____

Food & Hydration:_____

_____

_____

_____

Medical appointments, procedures or notes: _____

_____

DATE_____

Blood Pressure sitting ____/____ standing ____/____ Pulse _____BPM

Blood Sugar _____ **Menstrual cycle phase** __pre __pms __have period

Today I physically feel:

_____

_____

*Today I mentally feel:*_____

_____

Any unusual activity or events: _____

_____

Food & Hydration:_____

_____

_____

Medical appointments, procedures or notes: _____

_____

DATE_____

Blood Pressure sitting ____/____   standing ____/____   Pulse _____BPM

Blood Sugar _____   **Menstrual cycle phase** __pre   __pms   __have period

Today I physically feel:

_____

_____

*Today I mentally feel:*_____

_____

Any unusual activity or events: _____

_____

Food & Hydration:_____

_____

_____

_____

Medical appointments, procedures or notes: _____

_____

DATE_____

Blood Pressure   sitting ____/____   standing ____/____   Pulse _____BPM

Blood Sugar _____   **Menstrual cycle phase** __pre __pms __have period

Today I physically feel:

_____

_____

*Today I mentally feel:*_____

_____

Any unusual activity or events: _____

_____

Food & Hydration:_____

_____

_____

_____

Medical appointments, procedures or notes: _____

_____

DATE_____

Blood Pressure sitting ____/____ standing ____/____ Pulse _____BPM

Blood Sugar _____ **Menstrual cycle phase** __pre __pms __have period

Today I physically feel:

_____

_____

*Today I mentally feel:*_____

_____

Any unusual activity or events: _____

_____

Food & Hydration:_____

_____

_____

Medical appointments, procedures or notes: _____

_____

DATE_____

Blood Pressure sitting ____/____ standing ____/____ Pulse _____BPM

Blood Sugar _____ **Menstrual cycle phase** __pre __pms __have period

Today I physically feel:

_____

_____

*Today I mentally feel:*_____

_____

Any unusual activity or events: _____

_____

Food & Hydration:_____

_____

_____

Medical appointments, procedures or notes: _____

_____

DATE_____

Blood Pressure sitting ____/____   standing ____/____   Pulse _____BPM

Blood Sugar _____   **Menstrual cycle phase** __pre __pms __have period

Today I physically feel:

_____

_____

*Today I mentally feel:*_____

_____

Any unusual activity or events: _____

_____

Food & Hydration:_____

_____

_____

_____

Medical appointments, procedures or notes: _____

_____

DATE_____

Blood Pressure sitting ____/____ standing ____/____ Pulse _____BPM

Blood Sugar _____ **Menstrual cycle phase** __pre __pms __have period

Today I physically feel:

_____

_____

*Today I mentally feel:*_____

_____

Any unusual activity or events: _____

_____

Food & Hydration:_____

_____

_____

Medical appointments, procedures or notes: _____

_____

DATE_____

Blood Pressure sitting ____/____   standing ____/____   Pulse _____BPM

Blood Sugar _____   **Menstrual cycle phase** __pre __pms __have period

Today I physically feel:

_____

_____

*Today I mentally feel:*_____

_____

Any unusual activity or events: _____

_____

Food & Hydration:_____

_____

_____

_____

Medical appointments, procedures or notes: _____

_____

DATE_____

Blood Pressure sitting ____/____   standing ____/____   Pulse _____BPM

Blood Sugar _____   **Menstrual cycle phase** __pre __pms __have period

Today I physically feel:

_____

_____

*Today I mentally feel:*_____

_____

Any unusual activity or events: _____

_____

Food & Hydration:_____

_____

_____

_____

Medical appointments, procedures or notes: _____

_____

DATE_____

Blood Pressure sitting ____/____   standing ____/____   Pulse _____BPM

Blood Sugar _____   **Menstrual cycle phase** __pre __pms __have period

Today I physically feel:

_____

_____

*Today I mentally feel:*_____

_____

Any unusual activity or events: _____

_____

Food & Hydration:_____

_____

_____

_____

Medical appointments, procedures or notes: _____

_____

DATE_____

Blood Pressure   sitting ____/____   standing ____/____   Pulse _____BPM

Blood Sugar _____   **Menstrual cycle phase** __pre __pms __have period

Today I physically feel:

_____

_____

*Today I mentally feel:*_____

_____

Any unusual activity or events: _____

_____

Food & Hydration:_____

_____

_____

_____

Medical appointments, procedures or notes: _____

_____

DATE_____

Blood Pressure   sitting ____/____   standing ____/____   Pulse _____BPM

Blood Sugar _____   **Menstrual cycle phase**   __pre   __pms   __have period

Today I physically feel:

_____

_____

*Today I mentally feel:*_____

_____

Any unusual activity or events: _____

_____

Food & Hydration:_____

_____

_____

_____

Medical appointments, procedures or notes: _____

_____

DATE_____

Blood Pressure sitting ____/____ standing ____/____ Pulse _____BPM

Blood Sugar _____ **Menstrual cycle phase** __pre __pms __have period

Today I physically feel:

_____

_____

*Today I mentally feel:*_____

_____

Any unusual activity or events: _____

_____

Food & Hydration:_____

_____

_____

_____

Medical appointments, procedures or notes: _____

_____

DATE_____

Blood Pressure   sitting ____/____   standing ____/____   Pulse _____BPM

Blood Sugar _____   **Menstrual cycle phase** __pre __pms __have period

Today I physically feel:

_____

_____

*Today I mentally feel:*_____

_____

Any unusual activity or events: _____

_____

Food & Hydration:_____

_____

_____

Medical appointments, procedures or notes: _____

_____

DATE_____

Blood Pressure   sitting ____/____   standing ____/____   Pulse _____BPM

Blood Sugar _____   **Menstrual cycle phase** __pre __pms __have period

Today I physically feel:

_____

_____

*Today I mentally feel:*_____

_____

Any unusual activity or events: _____

_____

Food & Hydration:_____

_____

_____

_____

Medical appointments, procedures or notes: _____

_____

DATE_____

Blood Pressure sitting ____/____ standing ____/____ Pulse _____BPM

Blood Sugar _____ **Menstrual cycle phase** __pre __pms __have period

Today I physically feel:

_____

_____

*Today I mentally feel:*_____

_____

Any unusual activity or events: _____

_____

Food & Hydration:_____

_____

_____

Medical appointments, procedures or notes: _____

_____

DATE_____

Blood Pressure sitting ____/____   standing ____/____   Pulse _____BPM

Blood Sugar _____   **Menstrual cycle phase** __pre __pms __have period

Today I physically feel:

_____

_____

*Today I mentally feel:*_____

_____

Any unusual activity or events: _____

_____

Food & Hydration:_____

_____

_____

_____

Medical appointments, procedures or notes: _____

_____

DATE_____

Blood Pressure sitting ____/____ standing ____/____ Pulse _____BPM

Blood Sugar _____ **Menstrual cycle phase** __pre __pms __have period

Today I physically feel:

_____

_____

*Today I mentally feel:*_____

_____

Any unusual activity or events: _____

_____

Food & Hydration:_____

_____

_____

Medical appointments, procedures or notes: _____

_____

DATE_____

Blood Pressure sitting ____/____ standing ____/____ Pulse _____BPM

Blood Sugar _____ **Menstrual cycle phase** __pre __pms __have period

Today I physically feel:

_____

_____

*Today I mentally feel:*_____

_____

Any unusual activity or events: _____

_____

Food & Hydration:_____

_____

_____

_____

Medical appointments, procedures or notes: _____

_____

DATE_____

Blood Pressure   sitting ____/____   standing ____/____   Pulse _____BPM

Blood Sugar _____   **Menstrual cycle phase** __pre __pms __have period

Today I physically feel:

_____

_____

*Today I mentally feel:*_____

_____

Any unusual activity or events: _____

_____

Food & Hydration:_____

_____

_____

_____

Medical appointments, procedures or notes: _____

_____

DATE_____

Blood Pressure   sitting _____/_____   standing _____/_____   Pulse _____BPM

Blood Sugar _____   **Menstrual cycle phase** __pre __pms __have period

Today I physically feel:

_____

_____

*Today I mentally feel:*_____

_____

Any unusual activity or events: _____

_____

*Food & Hydration:*_____

_____

_____

_____

Medical appointments, procedures or notes: _____

_____

DATE_____

Blood Pressure sitting ____/____ standing ____/____ Pulse _____BPM

Blood Sugar _____ **Menstrual cycle phase** __pre __pms __have period

Today I physically feel:

_____

_____

*Today I mentally feel:*_____

_____

Any unusual activity or events: _____

_____

Food & Hydration:_____

_____

_____

Medical appointments, procedures or notes: _____

_____

DATE_____

Blood Pressure sitting ____/____ standing ____/____ Pulse _____BPM

Blood Sugar _____ **Menstrual cycle phase** __pre __pms __have period

Today I physically feel:

_____

_____

*Today I mentally feel:*_____

_____

Any unusual activity or events: _____

_____

Food & Hydration:_____

_____

_____

_____

Medical appointments, procedures or notes: _____

_____

What I have learned this month

_____

_____

_____

_____

_____

_____

_____

_____

_____

_____

_____

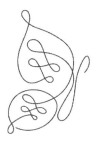

Things I have learned

By now, you have probably noticed some trends, and even figured out how to remedy them! In these pages, you can jot down the things you have noticed and if you haven't yet implemented changes into your lifestyle to help prevent pre-crisis or crisis, writing your thoughts on paper can sometimes open our eyes to things we haven't noticed before, and spark some ideas for what can later seem like obvious ways to prevent 'bad days.' You can also use these pages to discuss your findings with your health practitioner for other ideas on how to implement prevention.

Blood Pressure.
Make notations on what affects your blood pressure. Do certain events, foods, illnesses, or events over a few days make your blood pressure rise? Does it make it drop? How long does this last? Does it lead up to a crisis? Does your blood pressure drop when you stand up? Make any notations on your blood pressure as well as pulse! Always record your pulse along with your blood pressure. Is you BP low and your pulse high, or is your BP high and your pulse low? All of these things are important to tell your health care provider. Go back through your journal if you haven't noticed these changes and symptoms over the last year, and analyze your notes.

_____

_____

_____

_____

_____

_____

_____

_____

_____

_____

_____

_____

_____

_____

_____

_____

_____

_____

_____

_____

_____

_____

Blood Sugar. Make notations on what affects your blood sugar.

Do you feel emotional, moody, etc. if you need to eat? If so, is this confirmed with your blood sugar measurements? Do you get tired in the afternoon if you've eaten sugar or breads? And most importantly, Do repeated instances of low blood sugar precede a crisis or pre-crisis? Be sure you record the feelings/symptoms along with blood sugar numbers. If you don't have a meter, record whether low blood sugar symptoms are eased by eating, by eating proteins instead of sugars and carbs, or when you updose steroids.

_____

_____

_____

_____

_____

_____

_____

_____

_____

_____

_____

_____

_____

_____

_____

_____

_____

_____

_____

_____

_____

_____

_____

_____

_____

_____

_____

_____

_____

_____

_____

_____

_____

_____

Menstrual Cycle. Make notations regarding your

menstrual cycle. ... notes on regularity, PMS, heaviness, length, etc. Make notations if these factors coincide with any other symptoms, and/or with crisis or pre-crisis.

_____

_____

_____

_____

_____

_____

_____

_____

_____

_____

_____

_____

Feelings. Make notations on what you've discovered about the way

you feel and how it relates to your physical health. Do certain physical abnormalities indicate a crisis is coming? That you're getting dehydrated? Do certain illnesses make you head towards crisis unless you updose? Do you notice that if you're getting low on cortisol, or aldosterone, that you become irritable, moody, or depressed? Are you closer to crisis if you are experiencing brain fog, etc.? All of these things are extremely important to note and to have your family or those who are around you frequently watch for these things. These are all symptoms that can mean you need to pay attention to them!

_____

_____

_____

_____

_____

_____

_____

_____

_____

_____

_____

_____

Food & Hydration.   Make notations on how foods affect

you. Do any of them affect blood pressure, blood sugar, cortisol, dehydration? ANYthing you have noticed regarding food is especially important. Food and hydration affects our electrolyte status, and as we know, aldosterone controls water, sodium and potassium. Some foods lower cortisol, and caffeine is a diuretic which causes dehydration and loss of electrolytes. Make ANY notations on how you've discovered food affects your health and even moods – which in turn, affects cortisol.

_____

_____

_____

_____

_____

_____

_____

_____

_____

_____

_____

Meds & Supplements.   Make any kind of notation

regarding your medications and supplements, and how they affect you. Have you found that
maybe you'd be better off splitting up your steroids? Do certain medications make you bloat?
Have you added any supplements that changed how you felt, wither good or bad??
Note ANY changes or things you have noticed, and discuss with your practitioner.

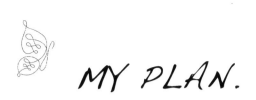

MY PLAN.

Based on the things you have learned this year, what is your plan for your care and to have a better quality of life? Be thoughtful and honest, and use this as a template for a discussion with your health practitioner.

_____

_____

_____

_____

_____

_____

_____

_____

_____

_____

_____

_____

_____

_____

_____

_____

_____

_____

WORKING WITH MY HEALTH PRACTITIONER.

After discussing your plan with your health practitioner, record your final plan that was made in conjunction with your health practitioner. This will serve as both a reminder and affirmation to yourself, and also an excellent source of information for your family, friends and emergency personnel should they need to reference it. Be sure and date it.

_____

_____

_____

_____

_____

_____

_____

_____

_____

_____

_____

_____

_____

_____

_____

_____

Changes.
Record any changes here that may be made after your health plan. Changes in medication, food/hydration, etc. Be sure to date it.

_____

_____

_____

_____

_____

_____

_____

_____

_____

_____

_____

_____

_____

_____

_____

_____

_____

_____

_____

Congratulations!

You have made an extremely committed and important start at being in control of your everyday health, educating and informing family, friends and health personnel, and in discovering how your body works and reacts to your Adrenal Insufficiency. This workbook has taken you through a microscopic look at each day for a year, records important information for you and others to reference, and helped you develop a plan with your health practitioner on living a better quality of life.

I am proud of you!!!! Use this space to write yourself a pat-on-the back, and feel proud of yourself!

_____

_____

_____

_____

_____

_____

_____

_____

_____

_____

_____

_____

_____

Made in the USA
Las Vegas, NV
25 November 2024